'Funny, you don't look like a Diabetic!'

JANET WATERSTON

'Funny, you don't look like a Diabetic!'

ASHGROVE PRESS, BATH

First published in Great Britain by
ASHGROVE PRESS LIMITED
Unit 7, Locksbrook Road Estate, Bath BA1 3DZ

A CIP catalogue record for this book
is available from the British Library

ISBN 1–85398–070–6

Photoset in 10½/12pt Palatino by
Ann Buchan (Typesetters), Middlesex
Printed by Redwood Books, Trowbridge, Wiltshire

Contents

Foreword

Diabetes is really two diseases. There is the medical part of the illness which is highly visible especially in hospitals or clinics and consists of insulin injections, blood tests and all the paraphernalia of diabetes. The other side of diabetes is secret and internal. It takes in the individual and highly personal emotions experienced by people with diabetes and those close to them. Although it is hidden and hard to measure, this internal diabetes governs the medical 'outer' part of the disease. If a person has a good relationship with their internal diabetes, they can live with it on reasonably good terms. If not, the diabetes often ends up ruling (and sometimes ruining) their lives.

Janet Waterston is someone who has a very good relationship with her own diabetes. This book is the fruit of her experience and commitment which she wants to share with others. In particular she concentrates on the importance of physical fitness as a way of building up self-esteem. I recommend this book to anyone involved with diabetes who wants to improve their understanding of this disease and find out how to deal with it in a positive way.

DR CHARLES FOX
Consultant Physician

To my mother Pierrette, and my husband Sean,
for their never failing love and support.
To the many individuals with diabetes, their
families, their friends and their health care teams.

PART I

Reviewed by
DR CHARLES FOX
Consultant Physician

1

Introduction

Hi! My name is Janet Waterston. I don't have a string of degrees, I'll never be a rocket scientist or a world class athlete. I'm just 'Joe average' and I happen to have diabetes.

I was diagnosed as having Type 1 diabetes when I was 12 years old, 19 years ago. That's more than half of my lifetime, including my radical teens and young adulthood. Over the years I've been through most of the ups and downs involved and I've learned a lot along the way.

I've spent over a year researching for this book, meeting and listening to hundreds of other people with diabetes discuss their major concerns and fears about having diabetes. The consensus was that there was a great lack of information and acknowledgement of the roles that the psychological aspects and the physical fitness related aspects play in good diabetes management.

It's always been felt that the best people to teach about diabetes have been people with diabetes themselves. This book was written by me, with contributions from the hundreds of other people with diabetes I've met. In writing this book I hope to make it all a little easier for everyone with diabetes, their families and their friends. For the young and the not so young, the fit and the not so fit.

At the time of writing, all information in this book is accurate. It is a collaboration between myself, numerous health care professionals and individuals with diabetes and should never replace or override the advice you receive from your medical team.

2

Diagnosis

TAKE HEART – YOU ARE NOT ALONE

There are 120 MILLION people with a form of diabetes world-wide. You may have just been diagnosed as having diabetes. The chances are that you've never been admitted to hospital before; in fact, you're probably rarely ever ill. There are many different emotions you may be feeling. The more common questions asked are:

Why me? What have I done to deserve this? Will it go away? Did I get diabetes because I kissed Henry who also has diabetes? Was it because I was lying about not doing my homework? Is it because I was always so wicked to my little brother? Or is it because I ate too many sweets?

Well I have to say, it's none of the above. The simple fact is in Type I diabetics, the beta cells which produce insulin were attacked and destroyed by your own immune system. Your body needs insulin to function properly and, at present, the only way to do this is with insulin injections or an insulin pump. Initially it's all a bit overwhelming, the fact that you have a condition for which, at the present time, there is no cure. It's hard to take in that you are now dependent on a drug and certain amounts of food and exercise for the rest of your life. And if that's not enough to ruin your day, you quickly learn that if you don't take control of your blood sugar levels and daily routine, your health could worsen. There's that threat of the dreaded complications. It's a lot to take on board but with education, patience and time, you'll be able to do it.

Before you get totally discouraged think of how fortunate you are to have all of the modern advances of medicine to work with. Insulin was discovered in 1922 by Canadian doctors Frederick Banting and Charles Best. That's only 73 years ago! If you were diagnosed prior to this, chances were that you would not have lived longer than twelve months from diagnosis.

Upon diagnosis the different emotions that you will go through are part of what is known as the grieving process.

There are five stages to this process.

1 shock and denial
2 anger
3 depression
4 bargaining
5 acceptance

It's important to go through this process in order to accept diagnosis.

Initially you'll feel SHOCK, in that you can't believe that it's happened to you because you've always been so healthy. You might DENY it and insist that there must be a mistake with the blood test results. Denial is a very common emotion and sometimes lasts for years.

Diabetes can occur at any time and to anyone, as you have proved. Few people are ever prepared for this. If you feel ANGRY about having diabetes, don't suppress it. LET IT OUT. It's healthy to do this, it's not healthy to keep it all in. One way that you can do this is by talking about your feelings. You have every right to feel angry. It's OK to let others know how you feel. Tell your family and your friends but make sure they know why you're pissed off, that it's because of having diabetes and it's not because you're mad at them. In this instance you don't have to be the Rock of Gibraltar.

Later you might feel DEPRESSED, totally isolated, and grieve for the person you once were. The diagnosis of any life long disease gives you a sense of loss, a sense of loss for the 'free'person that you once were. If you feel that it is difficult for you to talk about your feelings with family or friends because you sense that they just don't understand, then meeting other people who have diabetes is a great alternative. The British Diabetic Association can put you in touch with individuals or groups (see Appendix).

I had diabetes for eight years before I met and got to know anyone else who had it. I would have saved myself a lot of anguish had I known how helpful it would have been. This is where the saying 'If I only knew then what I know now' comes in. Just to know that there were other people out there who had the same feelings and concerns about having diabetes would have helped.

I can honestly say that it's great to meet other people with diabetes. You'll often feel a natural bond because you know they can relate whole-heartedly to what you go through in having diabetes. This contact can be a great help as you can learn through their experiences, good and bad, and take solace in knowing that others have the same feelings, worries, doubts and fears about having diabetes: that you are not alone. You may even gain a new perspective on diabetes from someone who accepts it as a challenge and has learned how to control it instead of letting it control them.

The most important thing to do after diagnosis is to educate yourself about diabetes. Research has shown that the more you educate yourself, the better your adjustment to diagnosis will be, because you'll feel that you are in control. Read CURRENT literature, books, journals and magazines. It's a good idea to contact and register with the various diabetes associations and pharmaceutical companies that specialise in diabetes products. They can supply you with newsletters and a wealth of information. It's your turn to become a mini doctor, chemist, dietician, psychologist, nurse and physiotherapist.

This will take time and effort, so do it at your own pace. It won't always be easy. Having diabetes will be a learning process of educating and re-educating yourself. The reason why you should educate yourself as much as possible is because the majority of the fears you have will be unfounded. In this situation, 'ignorance is not bliss'. You might have a preconceived idea of what diabetes is all about before actually knowing the facts. The more you educate yourself, the more you will understand about your diabetes and the greater your success will be in managing with it for the healthiest lifestyle.

Take charge of your health and look at it as if it were a challenge. Stay positive and dig deep inside yourself, because we can all live full, productive and healthy lives.

Remember, you're in charge!

3

Coping

Despite following insulin, diet and exercise plans, your blood sugar control may still be poor if you are unable to cope with the psychological pressures associated with diabetes. Before I get into all of this, I must say that I've experienced all these emotions over the years and I've had my moments when I just haven't been able to cope with it very well. It came as a relief to learn that these emotions were normal and that many other people with diabetes felt the same way.

SETTING PRIORITIES – FIVE STEPS TO COPING WITH DIABETES

From: *Diabetes Forecast*, Vol. 40
Copyright © by the American Diabetes Assoc. Inc.
Noreen Papatheodoron

Most people with diabetes feel swamped by the demands put on them, but most of their problems arise because they try to do too much at once. They try to change the habits of a lifetime overnight or attempt immediately to follow through every suggestion that the doctor has made. A better approach is to set priorities and to take things one at a time. This can be done by following the 'five C's'.

CLARIFYING with your health-care team what is most important for you.

CHOOSING from the health-care team's recommendations the goals or selfcare that are most important to you (e.g. weight loss, lower blood-sugar concentrations).

CHECKING that your goals are realistic, so that you do not programme yourself for failure.

CREATING an attitude of acceptance for the feelings of loss that come to you as you try to reach your goals (i.e. try to find out why you have had a setback and how you can prevent it happening again rather than criticising yourself).

CHANGING your long-standing habits so that you work your goals into your daily routines.

EMOTIONS

How you feel emotionally greatly affects your physical state and therefore your emotional well being is just as important as your physical state. Understanding the emotional aspects of diabetes is essential in accepting and effectively dealing with it. You may go through a full range of emotions after diagnosis. You might feel incompetent in not knowing what to do: how to adjust your insulin, plan an exercise programme, or even how to use a blood testing machine.

You might feel that your whole life has been altered; that you won't be able to live out your dream of travelling around the world with a backpack and tent or running a marathon. Don't be afraid of change or feelings of grief, it's a normal process. Incidentally, with the proper adjustments, you CAN live out these dreams and ambitions!

There is a lot of ANGER in having diabetes. After all, you didn't choose to have it . Why you, you ask? It really does seem unfair sometimes. I still ask that question of myself every once in a while.

GUILT is another strong emotion that you may experience. This relates to the feelings that you may have somehow failed or let yourself or others down. You feel guilty every time you eat a sweet or something that is not on your meal plan, you feel guilty if you don't test, don't exercise, or don't give your insulin on time. If that's not enough, others around you can make you feel guilty without realising that they are doing this. Your parents or partner can make you feel like this for not testing when THEY want you to, or for not exercising because you just don't feel like it. This may not make sense, but it is very common. Another person with diabetes summed it up by saying 'feeling guilty that you're doing something wrong is as much a part of the condition as is the medication.'

You need to balance your needs as a human being as well as the needs imposed by having diabetes. Once you have identified why you are feeling the way you are, you can take the appropriate steps to combat any negative emotions you may have.

It is not unusual to experience DEPRESSION after diagnosis. There is a lot to take on board and it can all seem pretty scary and isolating and sometimes you might just feel like giving up. It's very frustrating when you try your best to stay in good blood sugar control but you still can't get it right.

This is where educating yourself comes into play. You will learn that there are many variables involved in obtaining good blood sugar control. Some of these variables are out of your hands. For instance, if your are a teenager, you have active hormones to contend with. You should expect physical changes as well as mental changes to take place and interfere with your diabetes control. This can leave you feeling ' down and out'. Eventually this will alter and your diabetes control won't be so erratic. Remember, it's normal to feel discouraged at times, EVERYONE has their bad days as well as their good days.

STRESS

There is a connection between psychological stress and poor blood sugar control. The way that stress affects diabetes is a very individual thing. For most, it causes their blood sugars to rise and for others, it can lower it. The medical reasoning behind this is that stress triggers the production of hormones called, you guessed it, 'stress hormones' which cause the liver to release stored glucose to the body . If you are unprepared for this, your blood sugar will rise because there is not enough insulin and your body is unable to let the glucose into the cells where it can act as fuel.

There are two types of stress:

Positive stress : graduation, pay rise, marriage, winning the lottery, being in a sweet shop when your blood sugar is low.

Negative stress: failing an exam, arguing with someone, or God forbid, being stood up on a blind date when you know they saw you.

Contrary to what some people may believe, stress does not cause diabetes. Medical research states that a stress factor may simply have triggered the onset of diabetes and that you already had an underlying beta cell deficiency which made you more susceptible to getting it.

With time and practice, you will learn how the different types of stress affect your blood sugars and you'll be able to make adjustments accordingly.

Stress in the form of REBELLION may occur, especially as a teenager. You are asked to diet, test your blood sugar etc. and this could give you more reason to rebel as you'll have more to rebel about. Certain types of rebellion are not OK: not taking your insulin, not eating, being irresponsible and driving when your blood sugar level is low, or taking illegal drugs. If you want to rebel, there are plenty of other areas to rebel in: music, style of dress, hair and make-up. This is a less self-destructive and a healthier attitude to adopt.

MOOD SWINGS: Blood sugar levels can have an effect on how you feel. High blood sugars can make you feel frustrated, edgy, angry and sometimes downright horrid. Low blood sugar levels tend to make you feel sad, depressed, upset, quiet and hopeless. Fortunately, this is only temporary and once you have adjusted your blood sugar level, you are back to your old self. For some, this is just as unpleasant, with or without diabetes.

ADJUSTING AND ADAPTING

How you feel about having diabetes will change over the years. When you are younger you just want to fit in like everybody else. You tend to think that you are indestructible, that nothing can really harm you, or be that serious. So you don't take the threat of long term complications too seriously. You're more concerned with what you'll be doing next weekend and not how your health will be in 30 years from now. As you get older and have a better understanding of diabetes, your immediate concerns will change.

Much of our learning comes from trial and error through our own day-to-day experiences. We learn from the good and the bad times. Diabetes is a very personal affair, it affects everyone differently, both physically and mentally. Somebody else's way of coping may not be as effective for you and at the same time, their insulin doses and routines will not have the same effect on your control.

The only way to adjust and deal with all aspects of diabetes is by experimenting and experiencing. You can do this by using the information you've obtained from your doctors/ or diabetes nurse specialists, diabetes books and journals as GUIDELINES to follow. Another resource for learning is from meeting with other people who have diabetes and learning from their experiences. You'll find out how they've handled certain situations with their diabetes care. (Make sure they have followed a positive approach and not a negative one, as their course of action may not have been the right way!)

The three most difficult aspects of diabetes care to adjust to are: ongoing diabetes management, unpredictable swings in blood sugars, restrictions to diet. It can all be rather frustrating, even when you do everything right and it still doesn't guarantee a perfect blood sugar reading.

You can't take a vacation from having diabetes, you can't take a day off. Sometimes taking care of your diabetes is just PLAIN BORING! So, it does get a bit tiresome at times.

Adjustment and adaptation takes time and hard work but you CAN DO IT with the right attitude.

ATTITUDE

Some people take on the attitude that diabetes will kill them, therefore they must live life to the MAX right now! They indulge in dangerous sports, or go on binges of poor control, disregarding diet and insulin. It's almost like tempting fate. They think that their future looks so bleak and take the attitude of 'I'm going to be blind or develop kidney disease so why should I bother to take care of myself now?'.

Rather than dwelling on the negative, think of the positive aspects, which far outweigh them. The life-style we've adopted gives us a healthier advantage over other people who don't have diabetes and don't treat their bodies with the same self-respect.

Since we take better care of ourselves, we'll live healthier and longer lives.

– regular exercise
– well-balanced diet
– moderate alcohol intake
– daily foot care
– regular medical check-ups and monitoring
– no smoking
– regular rest

A sense of achievement and pride should be felt in what you are able to do. How many people do you know who could give themselves daily injections and blood tests?

Others feel the need to over-compensate because they have diabetes. It gives them that extra drive. If you channel this drive correctly, in a positive way, you can discover new avenues which you probably would not have sought out if you didn't have diabetes. e.g. participating in a triathlon or a marathon. You'll feel the greatest sense of accomplishment after completing one of these events. If this drives you, it's important to do this for YOURSELF and not for others. Don't feel that you have to prove anything to anybody. Just do it for yourself, because you want to.

Having diabetes also teaches us responsibility, self-discipline, and self-control. It gives us a sense of confidence in that we've 'overcome' another hurdle in life.

'SUCCESS ISN'T ONLY MEASURED BY WHAT WE HAVE ACCOMPLISHED, BUT ALSO BY WHAT WE HAVE OVERCOME'

MOTIVATION

Staying motivated is not always easy, especially when you are young and feel invincible. It is difficult because the benefits of good control are not always immediate.

A good way to keep yourself motivated is to write down

your goals, short term and long term. Be specific about these goals and state the reasons you want to achieve them and what you need to do. Most importantly, be realistic with these goals and set yourself realistic time scales to meet them.

If you find yourself moving away from these goals, review what you have written. Make sure that you haven't set your goals too high, tried to do too much at once. It takes time and hard work to change habits and routines.

A great incentive to stay in control is so that when scientists discover a cure for diabetes, and they will, you'll be as healthy as possible.

PERFECT CONTROL?

There are MANY variables involved in attempting to control blood sugar. There will be influences that you cannot control. But rather than getting upset and striving for 'perfect control' (which is unrealistic) set yourself guidelines. If in general you feel good, and that includes the odd hypo and hyper, and your blood sugars are in a reasonable range, then you are doing fine.

You can have a blood test called a Haemoglobin A_1 (HbA_1) done at your clinic. This is an excellent test to determine what your overall blood sugar control has been like. The amount of HbA_1 in the blood depends on the average blood sugar level over the previous 2–3 months. This is a very objective test, as the result doesn't depend on other factors such as time of day, exercise taken and meals, but simply your average blood sugar levels. With this result your doctor is able to guide you further and you can both set targets. The test results can also make you feel confident, knowing that things are going well or, on the other hand, it can alert you to when things are not going well.

Luckily, we now have portable blood sugar monitoring kits which consist of: a blood letting device – with disposable lancets (for pricking your finger), blood sugar test strips, and a meter. These monitoring kits enable us to get immediate blood sugar readings, which allows for tighter control. They are convenient and simple to use and most importantly they are accurate when used correctly. Experiment with several different types at your clinic to find the most suitable one for you. When you first start to use the blood letting devices on your fingers, you may feel some discomfort, but before long, you won't even notice that you've just pricked your finger. For the least amount of discomfort remember to use the sides of your fingertips and not the flat part and frequently change the lancets (just as you would your needles) to keep them sharp. Once again experiment with different types of devices and you'll be sure to find one that suits you. I used to hate testing my blood sugar until I found a device that's virtually painless. It's not such a drag to test anymore, I'm able just to do it and then get on with things, whereas before I'd spend half my time just psyching myself up for the inevitable.

There are NO advantages to high blood sugars. People who have tight control of their blood sugars are healthier than the ones who don't. This has recently been proven by the results of the North American Diabetes Control and Complications Trial (DCCT). The research has shown that there is a link between blood sugar levels and diabetes related complications. Dr Kenneth Quickel, President of the Joslin Diabetes Center states 'This result constitutes the most important research development since the discovery of insulin, and its application can reduce the complications of diabetes by half.' Although the benefits are clear, the study also showed that with an intensified regime, you are at a greater risk of hypoglycemic reactions.

So now, for the first time, when doctors say 'good blood sugar control is very important to your long term health' they have the FACTS to back up this statement.

When I was growing up I can remember saying to myself after I left the doctor's office, 'Well, it's never actually been proven that tight control affects your chances of complications.

The good news about the DCCT results are that tight control may delay or even prevent any complications!

You'll need to experiment to get your's right. With experience and knowledge you'll learn what works for you and you'll be able to allow having diabetes to work into/with your life-style, rather than the other way around.

If you feel that you are experiencing too many problems with your blood sugar control then perhaps you just need to change your insulin type or timing of exercise. Talk it over with your health care team as you might just need to try a new routine. Your control will change over the years just as your insulin doses will change. What was suitable for you when you were 13 will not necessarily be suitable for you at 25.

Don't get too discouraged, eventually you'll get it right.

You owe it to yourself to take control.

4

It's a Family Affair

PARENTS

'When I was 18, my father was so ignorant that I could hardly stand to have him around. But by the time I was 21, I was amazed at how much the old man had learned in 3 years.'
Mark Twain

Diagnosis of diabetes will also affect your parents, brothers and sisters. You may not realise or believe this, but they will also go through the different emotional stages of acceptance after your diagnosis. Some parents may not be able to handle diagnosis immediately. Their feelings will change, given time and understanding.

It is common for them to experience guilt and disbelief that their child has diabetes. They might blame themselves, thinking that they caused it by a particular incident that happened before diagnosis; e.g. a divorce in the family, moving house. All of this can leave them unable to offer support and comfort initially because they may still be experiencing these negative feelings. Don't forget that they are as vulnerable as you are.

The most common parental reactions to diagnosis are:

– Disbelief and irrational thinking; failing to believe and understand that THEIR healthy child has diabetes.
– Resentment and rejection; blaming their child for presenting a problem and interfering with the smooth running of the family.

I have a friend whose father has diabetes and after my friend was diagnosed, his father refused to speak to him for 3 months.

He could not cope with the fact that his son also had diabetes. He felt that he was to blame for this.

By nature parents are very protective of their children, particularly mothers. They tend to take over and handle your diabetes management. Because good blood sugar control is so important, they find it difficult to let go and let you handle situations on your own. Over protective parents can undermine your confidence by not allowing you to take control of your diabetes and be independent.

On a positive note some parents will accept, albeit with grief, that their child now has diabetes and will take an attitude of determination to find out about it and to do the best to help you.

Parents find it difficult to step back and allow their children to make mistakes. Even though this is the only way that you will learn, they often use the threat of complications to get you to have better control over your blood sugars. Because parents often fear hypoglycemia, they are more likely to discourage you from participating in strenuous activities or events where they will not be present, e.g. sleep-overs and parties. I've been given some advice from a mother who says her guide is that she has a good memory and can remember that what her teenagers are doing is only what she did at their age. Keeping herself informed with what they are 'up to' and accepting it is a far healthier attitude than pretending that they are not doing it.

Your parents need to be reminded at times that you are only a normal, healthy, growing individual and that you will go off your 'diet', not want to test your blood sugar all the time, and that you will have high blood sugar readings as well as the low ones.

It's important for you to remember that your parents only mean well when they ask, and keep on asking, 'Have you tested? Have you brought your supplies? Do you have enough food with you? Have you had your snack?' and so on, and so on. It's only natural for parents to over-react sometimes. Remember, they are always only looking out for your best interest. You'd probably do the same if you were in their shoes.

It's just as important for your parents to educate themselves about diabetes as it is for you. Many of the emotional problems connected with diabetes are due to the lack of knowledge and lack of acknowledgement of the problems involved by the family. More than likely, what little knowledge they have on diabetes will come from someone they know who has diabetes, usually an elderly friend or relative that has Type II diabetes. The disadvantage of this is that their friends treatment is very different from yours, and your parents might expect you to follow the same. Also, if this person has long-standing neglected diabetes they may have several of the complications, as they would have been diagnosed in the era before all the advances we now have in diabetes care; e.g. home blood sugar monitoring. The thought of these same problems happening to their child is quite devastating for any parent, especially if someone in their family had diabetes and they witnessed their poor control and deteriation.

If parents educate themselves about diabetes they will realise and expect your blood sugar control to fluctuate and will learn how to make adjustments. It's important for them not to place too much emphasis on one blood sugar reading, but to look at the overall picture.

I can't stress enough that there will be some fluctuations out of your control because of the many variables involved, e.g. stress from exams, hormonal changes; and parents should be made aware of this so as not to keep putting the blame on you. They must also learn to recognise the differences in your mood swings from having a hypo to just having a temper tantrum. It's up to you to make your parents aware of this and that not all mood swings are attributed to your blood sugar levels. Also, on the other hand, both sides should remember to leave points which could cause arguements to AFTER meals, not before.

It is very helpful for parents to be involved with a diabetes group, whether through the BDA or their hospital clinic. Interaction with other parents and their children can be invaluable and it could prepare them for changes that you may go through. They will learn that they also are not alone with their feelings, fears, and anxieties about having a child with diabetes. They'll be able to talk about these feelings and share them with understanding parents, without criticism. This can provide great comfort for them once they see that these feelings are acceptable and normal when living with diabetes. Once your parents come to terms with these feelings they won't feel so weighed down with feelings of responsibility, guilt, and being alone in this situation. They'll be able to relax a bit, which in turn will have a positive effect on your outlook and your diabetes control.

MOTHERS AND FATHERS USUALLY END UP BEING PARTICULARLY PROUD OF CHILDREN WHO HAVE DIABETES

A PARENT'S PERSPECTIVE

Like all parents I know, I can vividly remember the day my daughter was diagnosed as having diabetes. She was 5 years old then, she is now 24. Her diabetes hasn't been my responsibility for some years now, she copes with it, she accepts it and she's happy. It has been a long process and when I look back over the years, not so easily achieved. I don't know what it's like to have diabetes, I only know what it's like for me – a Mum whose youngest child cannot remember life without diabetes. But I can be selfish and perhaps a little self-indulgent and write about my part in Bev's diabetes and my needs, trusting that there is understanding that I am well aware of the problems she has faced and may well have to face and that I have always tried to help and support her.

Diagnosis itself produced in me a whole range of emotions – shock, anger, denial, guilt, sadness, and grief. Bev went into hospital to have her insulin doses and diet worked out, during which time innumerable people in white coats tried to teach me all about diabetes but no one seemed to understand that I couldn't take it all in – I could only think of the rest of my daughter's life and above all, my fear of injecting her. I'd been told she wouldn't be allowed home until I could do it properly and so, as instructed, I practised into an orange for 12 days, my fears growing greater with each day. On day 13 I did it.

Parents of children with diabetes go through added stresses as they experience injecting a very young child, denying them sweets and many of the things children love to eat, dealing with awful hypos in the night, worrying when they are late home and when they first drive a car, the upset the first time a boy/girlfriend ends a relationship because he/she has witnessed a bad hypo. Many of these worries are ours as parents and are not necessarily the worries of our children.

I was taught about hypos, hypers, complications and diet and I don't think I took any of it in. The only thing I can really remember being told was that we shouldn't have thickened gravy and this was by a rather plump dietician – no, I think she was actually fat and I felt very angry with her. How dare she be fat and talk to me and my little girl about diet! Never the less she did say we shouldn't have thickened gravy and this presented me with what was to be the first of many conflicts.

I was brought up in the North and my mother taught me that the way to a man's heart was through his stomach and that meant good thick gravy with EVERYTHING! So my problem was should I look after my daughter properly with thin watery gravy or should I look after my husband and son properly and have good thick gravy.

For about 3 months we had the watery kind then I decided that a bit of thickening couldn't really make all that much difference, so we had and still have good thick gravy.

Diabetes has presented many conflicts and of course, many guilt feelings. Some years later my husband and I were divorced and I can't help wondering if the thin gravy played a part!

I remember when we were at the hospital after diagnosis and the doctor telling me that working out the diet and insulin doses was relatively simple. So as time went by with all its changes and ups and downs it didn't seem all that simple. I followed all the instructions and rules but she still had hypos and hypers and because of what the doctor told me of it 'being simple' I never thought that it could be anything other than me doing things wrong. So every time results were not good I felt guilty. It was a long time before I realised that diabetes wasn't simple and so the overriding feeling it produced in me was guilt for not doing it well enough.

I felt a tremendous responsibility for my daughter's health and well being. I don't think for me that feeling of responsibility has ever completely gone away – I'm no longer responsible for the management of her health. She is; but I still feel responsible for how well she copes with it and life with diabetes. Letting her go and letting her make her own mistakes, knowing that her diabetes control would probably suffer for a time, was probably the most difficult thing of all.

She now lives in a flat with a couple of girlfriends and pops in and out of the house frequently – especially if the cupboard is bare! As a family we've been through a lot together, we've learnt a lot from living with diabetes and grown closer together because of it. I'm proud of the way both my children have coped. Like all parents of young people I now sit back and watch them entering the big, wide world and I know when I look back over the years that I could have done some things better but I also know, and equally important my children know, that in bringing them up, living with diabetes, I did the best that I could at the time.

A LETTER TO PARENTS

After sixteen years of being a parent the one overriding awareness I have of diabetes is that it poses conflicts for all of us in the family, and so often Mum is torn in many different directions. Disputes over matters such as music, hair, and fashion are trivial compared to the difficulties many of us experience during adolescence. I remember well the stage where I merely asked my daughter to tidy her room. She accused me of picking on her because she had diabetes!

Adolescence, among many other things, means rebellion. Much better to rebel at 15 than at 35 and if you have diabetes it surely would be abnormal not to rebel against it. Surely not to have conflicts involving diabetes when it is unavoidably part of our lives would be deliberately avoiding a very important issue and this would mean a lack of communication between parents and youngster. No communication and no basis for a lifelong relationship. At least with conflicts you have to walk through them and you do come to know each other and oneself much better, so achieving a relationship of mutual love, friendship and understanding.

I've no magic answers but over the years I have received some good bits of advice:

– If diabetic control sinks for a couple of years it won't do any long term damage so relax a bit and learn to watch and support rather than insist on perfect control.
– When there are conflicts and battles try to put aside your feelings or at least don't let them show, even if you are hurt and angry, and actually listen to your daughter/son and how they feel. Don't judge, don't deny and don't be critical of those feelings. They are real and he or she needs to be able to talk about them.

by MRS. JENNY HIRST (a well adjusted mum) mother of Bev Hirst, 24 years old (post teens, a well adjusted daughter) who was diagnosed at age 5.

SIBLING RIVALRIES

You can also expect your brothers and sisters to go through different emotions after your diagnosis. They might start to feel resentful of you because of all the special attention that you've been getting. Like your parents, they won't understand about diabetes at first. It's a good idea to discuss it once in awhile as a team. Brothers and sisters often feel helpless in not knowing what they can do for you, so let them know how they can help out and get involved. For example if you're having a hypo ask them if they can make you a drink or something to eat.

If you feel any hostility towards your siblings you may be thinking 'Why did I get diabetes and not them?' The old 'WHY ME?' syndrome. Perhaps your brother or sister could not cope with having diabetes. Learn different methods to cope with these feelings. It really takes a special, strong individual to be able to handle it all.

DIABETIC FOR A DAY

I've recently heard of an excellent idea from North America.
In order for a friend or a relative to really understand what

it's like to have diabetes, they could follow a diabetes routine for a day or more.

What's involved is: 4 injections (of sterile water!) and 4 blood tests. One before each meal and at bedtime. Follow a meal plan throughout the day and complete an exercise session at a gym/home.

The theme of this idea is 'empathy'. It can teach the friend/relative a new level of respect and understanding of what it's like to have diabetes and the daily rigours that it involves.

By someone showing this much care, the individual with diabetes will be proud that you have chosen to do this for them.

5

Relationships

SOUL MATES

Being honest about diabetes is the best way to avoid problems. A SIMPLE explanation of the facts is the best idea.

It's important to have trusting and understanding friends. They should understand what happens during a hypo and know what to do in case you need a hand. Whether it is giving you sugar or leaving you alone to take care of it. Friends like to be helpful, but if they are unsure of what to do then they might panic.

Explain to them your early warning signs and the best way to treat a hypo. Tell them that you might very well deny having a reaction and refuse any assistance. Describe how you might react, emotionally and physically, because everyone reacts differently. The emotional side is important because if you are anything like me during a hypo, where I get into a bit of a state and become very sullen, then you will want them to understand that it has nothing to do with them and how you feel towards them. Then reassure them that you'll be fine as soon as you treat your reaction.

Don't ever ignore your diabetes. It is nothing to be embarrassed or ashamed of. Real friends care and want to share your feelings. Try to involve friends without pushing them to understand. If they take an interest and learn about diabetes, they will appreciate the concerns and frustrations that you may experience at times.

Friends who don't accept you having diabetes don't have your best interests at heart and these are the type of 'friends' that you can do without.

KINDRED SPIRITS
(Significant Others)

Having diabetes doesn't stop someone from loving you, though it can make life a little more difficult at times. At least it's never boring!

Your partner must accept and understand your diabetes fully. As he or she will be one of your greatest influences.

Sometimes coping with diabetes can lead to reduced self esteem. It can make you feel insecure in that you might think that your partner will leave you for someone that doesn't have diabetes. Then he or she wouldn't have to worry or even think about all that is involved in living with someone that has diabetes.

I'll never forget how I felt the day my boyfriend started a new 6 month rota as a junior doctor. I was feeling a little unsettled as I had just moved to England and said good-bye to my family and friends and the great life-style I had in Vancouver, Canada.

As it turned out, the new rota my boyfriend was due to work on was in general medicine, which included the diabetes clinic at St. Marys Hospital. I was so worried that after his shift each day he'd come home and tell me that he didn't want to be with me anymore. I felt so insecure because working on this ward he saw all of the WORST cases with all of the advanced complications of diabetes. Albeit the majority of these patients were elderly with Type II, it didn't ease my conscience. So I got a little paranoid. I even went so far as to hiding my used test strips at the bottom of the dust bin so as not to remind him that I had diabetes and would ever be like the patients across the road in the clinic.

Well, I'm pleased to say that we survived that 6 month rota and I was even able to teach him, the doctor, a thing or two about diabetes.

Learning to live with something like diabetes can make you realise how important your relationship is to your partner. It can make you closer as you work together through the ups and downs. It's also a good indication of what the other person wants from the relationship. If they are willing to help and support you, they will stand by you.

There's no reason to change your habits for good blood sugar control to fit in with someone else's life-style either. A girl I know was just starting to date a guy she'd had a crush on for years. When they'd go out together she would purposely keep her blood sugars high so she wouldn't have to deal with a hypo and also, she didn't want him to see a change in her moods caused from having a hypo. He was a big, famous sports celebrity and she felt he could get any girl so she didn't want her diabetes to get in the way, by making her seem less of a catch. Eventually the relationship ended, not because of her diabetes, but with time she saw through his razz-a-ma-tazz, among other things. It was then she realised he never once asked about her diabetes, even after she finally told him she had it.

She's happier now and thankfully back in control with her blood sugars and realises that she was doing herself more harm than good. She also learned that that type of person was not good enough for her. She's now met a guy with the right attitude, he's involved and understanding, just as she is with him.

Don't ever blame your diabetes for the termination of a relationship. It's a convenient excuse and an easy way out. Just remember, it's his or her loss and certainly somebody else's gain!

A very common question is where, when and how do I tell my boyfriend/girlfriend that I have diabetes? This is a very individual thing. You choose when and how to tell someone. It's best to tell them early on in the relationship. There's no point in feeling that you have to hide it. At the same time, don't make a huge deal out of it. There's no need to recite your 'Living With Diabetes' manual as it will most certainly be too much for them to comprehend on one date. Remember how its been a constant learning process for you also.

Wearing an I.D. Medic Alert bracelet can come in handy in this situation as it can be a starting point for discussion on diabetes.

LOVING DIABETES
by Peter Welsh

I met Joanna in 1970, at a University motor club 'squash for freshers'. I was the fresher. She had a London degree and was married to a post-grad. He had a beard. I thought she was terribly together and so unattainable that the issue of whether I was actually attracted to her could not even be contemplated.

We were part of a Cambridge set who learned a lot about motor sport, a bit about life, and absolutely nothing of any academic significance. Joanna's husband was a bright immunologist who appeared to have proprietary rights over her blood chemistry. He seemed far more involved in it than she was.

I don't remember when I became aware that she had diabetes. I didn't know anything about it except that you had to have injections. I had worked in a garage belonging to my uncle, and his partner, George Johnson, had diabetes. George was a tall quiet man who taught me how to service Morris Minors, and who retreated into the loo to do mysterious and apparently slightly unwholesome things.

My clearest memory of Joanna's diabetes at University arises from a trip a group of us made to watch the RAC Motor Rally. We went to Yorkshire, to a special stage which finished halfway up a notorious Sutton Bank, a one-in-four hairpin climb from the Vale of York to the North York Moors. It was a November midnight with a freezing, howling, white-out blizzard causing chaos among competitors and spectators alike. It was less than 300 yards from the shelter of the tree-line to our cars parked at the top of the bank, but in this distance we were all frozen and buffeted mindlessly by the ferocity of the storm.

Joanna seemed particularly affected and her husband (through a beard of ice crystals) talked about a 'hypo'. At that time I didn't know what this was. Looking back, I thought it more likely to have been hypothermia, rather than hypoglycaemia.

In due course I graduated, and took up gainful employment to pay for my expensive tastes in motor racing. I stayed in touch with Joanna and her spouse. In fact, I held their relationship in some awe, as a model of marriage. I was accordingly devasted when she left him, and erotically bemused when she and I became lovers.

But she went back to him, and I married someone else. Over the next few years our paths wove in and out, at times close and at times distant, until, with a certain inevitability, we were drawn back together by the almost palpable bond which vibrates between us. We now live together in an old coal merchant's house; me, Joanna, and diabetes.

So what's it like, living with diabetes, for me the very first thing that occurs to mind is FOOD. As far as I'm concerned diabetes is all good news here. As I grew up, my basic approach to food was to eat a lot of what I liked, and as little as possible of what I disliked; both judged purely on the basis of smell, taste and texture. I was completely ignorant of the existence of protein, carbohydrates, fats, etc. I did have a profound belief that fish gave you brains and carrots helped you see in the dark but that was it in terms of dietary awareness. Since there is some history of heart disease in my male relatives, and I'm fairly heavily built (although beautifully proportioned), this amoral omnivorous approach would certainly have caused me real problems, even if I survived the scurvy.

Joanna's approach to food is very different to mine: much more informed, and if anything the results are better tasting as well! Another real bonus is the fact that she always has some tasty morsel concealed about her person, sometimes even a chocolate Hob-Nob which I can greedily devour! I still can't calculate at a glance the insulin needed for an Indian meal, as she can, but I now have a new and much more useful awareness of how to eat to really stay alive.

After food, I think the next impact of living with diabetes has been on my attitude to medicine, doctors and illness. I used to regard doctors as totally knowledgeable and completely infallible. I think many people do. Very slowly, by talking to Joanna and to other people with diabetes, I realised that a doctor's 'prescription' is not a magic elixir which will be effective, independent of the behaviour of the individual who receives it.

I also discovered that doctors are PEOPLE, who can be ignorant, wrong, or too busy to pay the necessary attention to the individual in front of them. I met the parents of a not-so-newly diagnosed teenager who had not understood, or had not been told, that the child's insulin dose could be changed. The family had endured crashing hypos until finally, in a kind of dazed desperation, they had gone to a BDA branch meeting and been encouraged back to their doctor to seek improved guidance.

With more than a little reluctance (it seemed too UNSCIENTIFIC) I eventually had to acknowledge that how I felt, emotionally, greatly affected my physical state. This is a practical reality for people with diabetes: Joanna's insulin requirements drop by almost half when she's relaxed and happy.

Hypo's don't worry me. Joanna has them occasionally, typically something like mid-afternoon when we've been strenuously decorating the house and she hasn't had quite enough lunch. She has pretty good warning signs. Usually whatever she's doing unaccountably gets very difficult and there is a lot of 's"t' type muttering under the breath. A Twix is usually called for and does the trick. It takes eight minutes of sitting doing not much and then her blood sugar comes back to something recognisable.

Night hypos are rare and, frankly hilarious. Often she won't wake and the only sign is a very heavy sweat. I do this as well and in my case the cure turns out to be a milky drink before sleep. I wonder how blood sugar levels in 'normal' people really do vary. However, sometimes she does stir, and then I'm treated to the most amazing upside-down conversation. She is completely authoritative, completely definitive, and completely incomprehensible. Usually no action on my part is needed and sleep soon descends. Very occasionally she does go very low and then I resort to glutinous, and literal, sweet talk to get her to eat a Twix, or whatever else is on duty at the bedside.

I don't like having injections myself. My own experience of them is limited to the routines of childhood, the dentist, and occasional anti-tetanus after injuries gained from motor racing. They hurt; me, anyway. Joanna is adamant that the fine needles on her NovoPen don't hurt at all, even when she's used one for a week and it's so blunt that the skin depresses half an inch before the needle penetrates. She injects in public which is fine with me, and I've never witnessed other onlookers having problems either. To be fair, I do recall a waiter at a Greek restaurant being so distracted that he walked into a pillar, but he wasn't actually OFFENDED.

I have met other people with diabetes who won't inject in public. I remember Joanna and I were once eating, together with a friend with diabetes, in a mobile home. Joanna had injected herself at the table when suddenly we heard this tremendous banging and shuffling. Our friend had retired to the tiny loo to inject himself, and had become entangled with the various undesirable objects which were stored in what was effectively a small (insanitary broom cupboard. Only the three of us were there and yet he still risked latrine entrapment rather than 'public' injection.

So far Joanna has never had any 'complications'. I drove her to her last eye test, so she could have her pupils dilated and not have to drive home herself. As she came out of the consulting room the specialist said in a very loud voice: 'Well, Joanna, your eyes are fine, no problems there at all'. I have never asked her, but I wonder if this was for my benefit? She's very careful with her feet and this taught me something else that somehow I'd mislearned. It is O.K. to take time to look after yourself. This is a difficult lesson to get right once you mislearn it. I've met more than one newly diagnosed, elderly non-insulin dependent diabetic, who had real problems with the idea that they needed to attend a little to their own well-being: neighbours, yes; grandchildren, of course; themselves, 'a nuisance'.

What's the downside to loving diabetes? I've tried hard to see one but honestly can't. Loving diabetes is much more to me than the few words written here, but I will try to sum it up in a sentence. I love Joanna; and she, with and without her diabetes, has taught me more about life and myself than anyone else I have ever met. I wouldn't have missed it for the world.

6

Independence

DRUGS

There is very little information on how illegal drugs can affect diabetes control. It's probably because no one wants to condone it, including myself.

However, since we are just like everybody else, some of us are bound to try. Whether you have diabetes or not, taking drugs is very harmful. It can be dangerously addictive.

Now if you still insist on experimenting with drugs there are certain precautions to take. Learning how illegal drugs affect your diabetes control may help you avoid too many problems.

CANNABIS: lowers blood sugar and increases your appetite which gives you the 'munchies'. This in turn will cause you to eat more and you know the effect that this has on your blood sugar (this can lead to hyperglycemia and make your diabetes harder to control). Other effects of cannabis are lethargy, confusion, and paranoia.

AMPHETAMINES: the effects are unlimited energy, nervous excitability and lack of appetite. So to someone who has diabetes this means using energy and lowering blood sugar, and with a lack of appetite you risk not being able to treat the hypo.

ECSTASY: the effects are euphoria, heightened sensual awareness leading to increased blood pressure and heart rate.

LSD: varies from mellowness to disorientation, dizziness, anxiety and violence which can all leave you feeling very confused and not knowing whether you are coming or going and forgetting or not caring about your blood sugar levels.

BENZODIAZEPINES (mild tranquillisers): effects are drowsiness, confusion, hostility, talkativeness and excitability. These reactions can make you confused as to whether you are having a hypo or suffering from high blood sugar.

COCAINE: it has an adrenalin-like effect and could increase your blood sugar and alter your eating habits. Your chances of having a heart attack are also increased.

STEROIDS: some athletes use this drug to make themselves huge. They can make muscles larger than natural. Steroids lower blood sugar levels and can make you very aggressive and withdrawn. They also increase your risk of blood vessel damage and heart disease.

Some of the greatest risks of taking drugs is that they can alter your consciousness, and sense of time and judgement. This could cause you to forget to take your insulin, test your blood sugar, forget to eat and make you unaware of low blood sugar symptoms. All of which could lead to a hypoglycemia or hyperglycemia reaction. Another thing to consider is the unreliability of street drugs. You might be getting something other than what you expect – which could really effect your diabetes control!

TOBACCO

'Every cigarette smoked is another nail in your coffin'

Dr. Robert Elkeles
(Consultant Physician, Diabetes Specialist)

Anti-smoking laws are getting stricter because the harmful effects of inhaling cigarette smoke, by smokers and non smokers, are being publicised more. Which is good news for people with diabetes as it has serious side effects to your long term health. Smoking leads to decreased circulation by narrowing small blood vessels. It also plays a major role in coronary heart disease, which is the leading cause of death in the U.K. Why add an extra burden by smoking? Especially since it is something that you can control.

It's important to realise that by smoking you are not only harming your health, but also the health of those close to you – and that is very selfish. Second hand smoke (passive smoking) also causes serious health problems.

It only takes less than half a pack of cigarettes to develop a nicotine addiction. This addiction is very strong which is why it is so difficult to give up.

A lot of people are afraid to give up smoking for fear of gaining weight, despite knowing of the serious health implications. It is known that you can develop a craving for sweets which in turn may cause some weight gain. Don't get discouraged if this happens because it is far better for you to put on a few pounds temporarily than to continue smoking and permanently harm your health. Once you rid yourself of the nicotine addiction it will be easier for you to lose the extra weight you may have put on.

ALCOHOL

This is a tricky one, but the golden rule to follow is: everything in MODERATION. Your social life shouldn't be affected by having diabetes. Just be sensible about it. Ask yourself if it's really worth it, to go out on a major drinking blitz, and then suffer the consequences the following day and very often for several days afterwards?

The best time to drink is with a meal, as alcohol lowers blood sugar, making a hypo more likely to happen. Alcohol also impairs your judgement and you may not realise that you are having a hypo. Often symptoms of a hypo are similar to that of being drunk. This can confuse friends who may not be aware that you are hypo and then not able to help you.

It's a good idea to test your blood sugar during the course of the evening and have a friend that knows how to do this as well. The tendency towards hypos can last for 4 to 6 hours after you drink. So make sure that you test before you go to bed.

Different types of alcohol affect your blood sugar in different ways. Dry white wine, shots of vodka, or gin on the rocks will lower it. Whereas champagne and orange juice, kahlua and milk, or Harvey Wallbangers will cause it to increase. You'll need to take note of the sugar content in certain drinks to enable you to take the appropriate precautions.

Alcohol is high in 'empty calories' (no nutritional value), therefore it's also very fattening. So if you want to lose weight, it's a good idea to stick with DC's (Diet Cokes) and have the odd glass of wine or beer.

HORMONAL CHANGES

Hormone – a substance produced within the body and carried by the blood to an organ which it stimulates. *Oxford Dictionary*
Growth Hormone – a hormone which stimulates the growth of bone and muscle mass during puberty.

Hormonal changes are two dirty words in diabetes control if you are a teenager.

Research shows that a hormone called Growth Hormone (GH), acts as an anti-insulin agent. This means that when your sugar level drops, it stimulates the release of adrenalin which triggers the release of stored blood glucose. The result of all of this is blood sugar levels that sway from too low to too high.

It can be very frustrating when you are trying hard to keep a balance. Especially if you have parents jumping all over you saying 'you are not taking care of yourself!'. When this happens, just remember that it's not all your fault and these uncontrollable blood sugars won't go on forever.

Hormonal changes aggravate diabetes making it harder to control. Because of this resistance to the effects of insulin, you will have to give larger doses of insulin. Taking more insulin doesn't mean that the severity of your diabetes is worse. Check with your doctor or nurse for guidelines for the correct doses.

During this stage of your life you want to be totally independent. You want to show that you can take control of yourself and your diabetes. It can be very frustrating when you've tried your best, have done your blood testing and stuck to a healthy diet, and your blood sugar levels still swing out of control. It's almost tempting to rebel, go on food binges, skip insulin injections, or refuse to test.

As a teenager the independence you crave for is more difficult to achieve with diabetes. There are conflicting demands between independence, wanting to be carefree with few responsibilities, and dependence, following a daily regime of diabetes management. The contradiction between the two can lead to resentment, and rebellion which can affect the relationship you have with your parents.

Recognise the limits of your control. The freedom and flexibility you want will come through knowledge and understanding of your diabetes.

REBEL YELL

All of the added responsibilities which are placed on us because we have diabetes make the stage of independence all that more difficult. We are forced to conform when all we want to do is rebel like all of the other kids on the block. This can lead to a lot of stress, especially as when we are teenagers we tend to make mountains out of mole hills. EVERYTHING becomes traumatic.

You are expected to conduct yourself in a mature, responsible fashion even though you have not fully developed emotionally and mentally. You are expected to make intelligent decisions even though your intelligence has not fully developed.

With your increased assertiveness at this stage, try not to use your diabetes as a weapon of rebellion against your parents and other adults. e.g. use hypos as a means to avoid something that you don't want to do. As tempting as this may be.

Having diabetes is like an intrusion at this stage. You'll need to find a balance of self-care and assistance from your parents and health care team.

Peer group pressure has such a strong influence at this time of our lives. The social scene of late night partying and boozing followed by a pizza binge at 3am doesn't exactly coincide with what doctors suggest for good diabetes management. We have to come to terms with the limitations that diabetes poses on us at times and learn how to make sensible adjustments to enable us to do what we want.

REBEL WITH A CAUSE

I was told that I had insulin dependent diabetes when I was nine years old. I lived with my mum and my grandparents who first noticed that I was ill.

For some time, I had been having terrible stomach pains and tiredness, and I had been losing weight. I had turned from a plump child into a slim one. For the first time in my life I could wear fashionable clothes instead of the tentstyle ones that I normally had to wear. I was also passing amazing amounts of urine, and drinking like a fish. I would come home from school and quickly finish off a two litre bottle of coke, which made my thirst worse.

I remember my grandmother forcing my mum to take me once again to visit the doctor and to demand tests. I'd been to the doctor five times, and each time he had either said that I had a chest infection, or that it was 'nothing to worry about'. This time we saw a different doctor and she tested my urine for glucose.

She tested it with some funny looking strips, waited, then announced that I was diabetic and would have to be admitted into hospital. My reaction was to sit and cry my eyes out.

I went into hospital, and learned how to deal with my diabetes. My family got used to living with it too, and for a couple of years everything was OK. Then in September 1983, I started secondary school. The first morning mum came with me, so she could be sure that the head of my house group knew that I had diabetes. He in turn told my teachers about how I would need to eat two snacks during the morning and afternoon. He gave me a card so I could remind the teachers about all this. Only one teacher, Mr Sims the science teacher, kept forgetting that I had diabetes.

Because I needed to inject twice daily, if a teacher gave me a detention they would discuss it with mum and agree for me to do the detention either during my lunch break or spread over the week. For example, a half hour detention would become 15 minutes for two days. At first my diabetes was a problem, but eventually my friends had got used to it and accepted me for what I was, and stopped acting as if they could catch diabetes from me (which is impossible). I had trouble from the school bullies calling me names, but when they realised that it didn't upset me anymore they stopped.

Making new friends at secondary school was easy. I had my old friends from junior school who knew about my diabetes, but I hid it from my new friends. I started eating my two snacks during break or I would ask to go into the toilet and eat them there. Everything was fine until I was admitted to hospital to have my insulin changed. Mr New, my form teacher, had told my form group why I was in hospital. When I returned to school, all my new friends treated me like the plague, so to get my friends back again I did something really stupid. I began to ignore that I was diabetic. At first I began to cheat on my diet – add an extra exchange here and there – then I started to eat Mars bars and drink sugary coke. I ate or drank these things during break times at school or as I walked home, so Mum wouldn't find out my secret. I ballooned up from seven stone to just over ten. I began to find ways of bringing the sweets and coke into the house and by 1986, my diabetes was wildly out of control. I just didn't care. For the first time since being told that I had diabetes I was enjoying myself. When I attended the diabetes clinic, Dr Young decided to re-admit me to hospital and start me on the NovoPen. However, once I had been released from hospital, my unruly behaviour towards diabetes didn't change. The final straw was when people began to comment on my weight. I needed to find a way to lose weight quickly. I thought that if I cut down the amount of insulin I injected I would lose at least a tiny bit of weight. In my mind I knew it was a stupid thing to do, but try reasoning with a head-strong teenager who wouldn't listen. I ended up in hospital four times in three months with ketoacidosis. No one knew what I was doing – the doctors at the hospital thought it was due to the stress of the mock exams I was taking at school. I finally did something really stupid. Because I was now on the NovoPen treatment I stopped injecting all three of the short acting insulin and only injected 28 units of Human Monotard. Eventually I did lose weight. I eventually weighed six and a half stone and began to suffer from diabetic complications, mainly retinopathy, which if left untreated leads to blindness.

In 1989, I finally stopped mistreating myself. After about six years of ignoring my diabetes, I took control of my life.

There is a moral to my story. No, it isn't 'stick to your diet or else you'll end up blind', etc. It's this. If you ever feel sick of being diabetic and begin to ignore it, stop and think about the risks. A blow out now and then isn't going to hurt anybody, as long as it isn't every week! Finally, remember this. Diabetes lives with you, you don't live with it. You should control it, not the other way round.

By Gina Wasley

SEXUAL IDENTITY

To develop a sexual identity you have to accept your own body. During our teens our body image is more crucial to our well-being than at any other time in our lives. Most people feel 'gawky' and 'imperfect' at this stage, with or without having diabetes.

With having diabetes we know that we are not 'perfect'. This can lead some people to ask if they'll be accepted by the opposite sex. This can cause low self-esteem and the fear of rejection. You might want to isolate yourself from your friends to protect yourself but this will actually be worse for your self-esteem. If you talk to your friends or just your best friend about these feelings, you'll realise that they'll have the same fears and insecurities, and that nobody is 'perfect'.

7

Men

A FRANK LOOK AT IMPOTENCE

Impotence is not inevitable to all men who have diabetes. It is common enough to cause concern, yet it is the least talked about of complications related to diabetes.

Before we go into this any further, let's take a look at what it all means. Impotence is defined as the inability to achieve or sustain an erection during sexual intercourse. Once aroused, the three spongy areas of the penis fill with blood and expand to cause an erection. This blood flow is controlled by the nervous system, nerves and blood vessels play a key role in this process. If someone has damage to the nerves or damage to the blood vessels, than the erectile function can be impaired.

There can be a number of causes of impotence in relation to diabetes:

– poorly controlled diabetes – potency should return to normal once blood sugar control has been resumed. (another motivating factor to stay well controlled)
– the onset of diagnosis or pre-diagnosis of diabetes – once treatment has commenced and blood sugars are controlled, this problem should be alleviated.
– nerve damage – the result of damage to the nerves that supply impulses to the pelvic area. These nerves control the erection reflex. This is the main organic cause of impotence. There is growing evidence that good blood sugar control can slow down damage to nerve and blood vessels.
– blood vessel damage – deterioration of large and small blood vessels carrying blood into and from the pelvic area.
– psychological – you might become so concerned about im-

potence happening to you that this could actually lead to stress, anxiety, and depression, which in turn could cause impotence.

– alcohol and drug abuse affect sexual function – you might freak out and worry thinking that you're impotent when you are unable to sustain an erection and make love to your babe at 3 am, after you've just completed a Guinness guzzling competition. Not to worry, alcohol has this affect on the majority of the male population. Diabetes or not. I suggest laying off the booze a little if you plan to do any rumba the night of a major party.

* Final note: sex is exercise so like every good Boy Scout: BE PREPARED . . . have your Lucozade handy.

THE FACTS

– Impotence is 3 to 5 times more common in individuals with diabetes than in non diabetics.

– An estimated 50–70% of the male population that have diabetes will never have to cope with long-term impotence.

– 20% of the male population (with or without diabetes) is impotent by the time they reach 60 years of age. In all men, the risk increases with age.

Impotence caused by diabetes comes on gradually rather than all of a sudden. It can take anywhere from months to years for it to fully develop. In other words, just because you weren't able to maintain an erection the last time you attempted to make love doesn't mean that you are now impotent. Don't freak out because there could have been a number of reasons involved. e.g. you had too much to drink, physically tired, stressed out due to work/exams.

If you have nocturnal erections, chances are that impotence is due to a psychological cause rather than an organic one.

The good news is that if you experience impotence, it's not all gloom n' doom. You can still have an active fulfilling sex life. In most cases the libido (sexual desire, drive) is not affected by impotence. There are various forms of treatment and counselling you can consider.

Talking about it is the first step towards treatment. Seeking advice from your GP or diabetes specialist can be very beneficial. They can advise you on all of the best options available to you. You might want to bring your partner with you as you are both in this together and you will both gain knowledge and understanding. There's no need to ever feel embarrassed or ashamed. The most important thing to do is to talk honestly and openly.

Communication with your partner is crucial here. There are a lot of emotions to consider when discussing impotence. It's important for your partner to understand that it is not because you no longer love them or don't find them attractive. Don't expect them to know what you are thinking and feeling. This is where WORDS speak louder than ACTIONS.

FERTILITY IN MEN

The nerves and blood vessels that are affected in impotence do not have an effect on fertility in the diabetic male.

8

Women

PREGNANCY

Back in the 1930s there was a 50% mortality rate for children of diabetic mothers therefore most women were discouraged from having babies.

Years ago I decided that I wouldn't have children because of the risks involved with having diabetes. I was afraid of all of the horror stories I heard about diabetic mothers and their HUGE babies.

Today, with the advances in modern medicine, a lot has changed. I'm happy to say that I've changed my mind and am now looking forward to starting my own family.

The chances of having a healthy baby are very optimistic these days. In order to maximise these chances there are a few ground rules to follow. These require dedication and commitment both to your health and to the health of your baby. Doctors say it is unfortunate that women don't exert the same control with their diabetes at other times. It is easy to say that you can't find a better motivating factor than knowing that your diabetes control directly affects your unborn child.

A good lesson to learn from this is that it will make you realise that you CAN achieve good diabetes control as long as you stay motivated.

THE PATH TO A BOUNCING BABY

Lynne Carney details the needs, actions and emotions associated with her first pregnancy.

We made the decision in January 1993 to start thinking about starting a family.

I've been diabetic since I was 21, so I had established my lifestyle and general approach to life insulin-andBM-stick-free, unlike Kevin, my partner, who was diagnosed at the age of 4. I've never been what you might call a particularly 'good' diabetic. I'd managed, don't get me wrong – my HbA_1's were generally around 9–10% at a hospital where normal non-diabetic levels were 8.5% – but this was more down to good luck than good management. In the January of 1993 I hadn't done any regular blood tests for around two years – just the occasional one to confirm my worst fears when the back of my throat began to feel like the bottom of a budgie's cage. So I knew I had a lot of hard work to do to regain control before hanging up the diaphragm and spermicide.

So, later that month I took myself off to see my Diabetic Liaison Health Visitor (or whatever her title is!), to discuss pre-conceptual care. She went through the type of diabetic control that is aimed for and why, the local system for medical care once I got pregnant, what I might expect from the birth and early child care and also gave me general fitness and health advice. She also gave me a blood test meter on long term loan which made the task of four/five tests per day somewhat easier to bear.

It is important that all women improve their general fitness levels before attempting to get pregnant, but it is particularly essential that diabetic women achieve good control before discontinuing contraception. The majority of limbs and organs are formed within the first eight weeks after conception – high blood sugars can disrupt this process leading to serious congenital disorders and malformation. If you take into account the fact that most women do not have pregnancy confirmed until six–eight weeks, it is vital that blood sugars are consistently kept as near normal as possible to ensure normal development of the embryo.

This obviously carries the implication that whilst you are trying for a baby, excellent control should be maintained at all times – not an easy job, particularly if it takes some time to get pregnant.

I started a regime of four blood tests per day, aiming at results between 4–8 mmol. It makes sense for any woman to prepare for pregnancy by improving diet and general fitness levels, however this is also an important factor in improving control. I cut down on alcohol, started doing some exercise on a reasonably regular basis (at least three times per week) tried to eat a few more fresh vegetables and fruit and cut back on convenience foods. Lots of good intentions – certainly the local pub profits dropped a bit, but with work demands and my general lassitude it wasn't easy to keep to it all. However my control did improve and I even lost a little weight over the next three months. In April we had a holiday in the sun – on the basis that it might be the last opportunity for some time to go anywhere quite so exotic! I had two weeks of eating and drinking myself daft! On our return I cracked down intensively and after a few more weeks decided that I was back in the driving seat, and gave up contraception. I'd not expected to feel so apprehensive, but after so many years of being so careful not to get pregnant abandoning contraception completely felt very strange and scary!

We settled in for a few months of disappointment and surely enough 4 days later along came a period. However that was the last one – it took only 3 weeks for me to conceive and by 4th June, with a period one day late, I was in the chemist buying pregnancy testing kits. The first test I did was negative. It was followed by a small amount of bleeding and I assumed we hadn't been successful, and opened and drank most of a bottle of wine. Mistake! I know now that until sufficient pregnancy hormones have built up, tests can give a negative result and that as the fertilised egg embeds in the lining of the uterus a small amount of bleeding can occur.

In actual fact I had conceived two weeks earlier and was at this point four weeks pregnant (the dates are calculated from the first day of the previous period – don't ask me why!). Two days later, with what I had thought was my period having disappeared entirely, I tested again – with a rather inconclusive result. Two days further on however there was no mistaking it – definitely two blue lines!

I rang the Health Visitor and was told to attend the Diabetic Ante-natal Clinic that Thursday.

Most non-diabetic women will not have their first antenatal clinic until c. 12–14 weeks. I had mine at 5 weeks and then attended once a fortnight until late in the pregnancy when it changed to once a week.

I found the fortnightly visits really helpful. I was performing blood tests four/five times per day and occasionally in the middle of the night. The Diabetes Specialist and Health Visitor would review my test results over the last two weeks with me, which meant problem areas were identified and dealt with promptly, and HbA_1 tests were performed once a month which gave me an overview of my control on a very regular basis. I also had the home phone numbers of the diabetes team should any problems arise in between appointments. This was complemented by fortnightly confirmation that the baby was growing normally and the opportunity to get to know the midwives and the hospital system – something that was invaluable later on!

Early on I had real problems with erratic high results – my regime was at this point a morning dose of Ultratard with three doses of Actrapid (by Novopen) before meals. The Ultratard was moved to bedtime, but this just moved the problems to a different time of day,. The Ultratard was then replaced with Protaphane (delivered at bedtime) which is apparently absorbed more evenly and this helped even out control somewhat. Over the whole pregnancy my dosages were constantly tweaked and adjusted to respond to my changing needs and I was positively encouraged to be responsive to any trends I could see emerging from my own knowledge – it felt very much that this was a team effort!

I was fortunate enough that I didn't suffer from morning sickness or nausea at all – just extreme tiredness which was really easy to cope with. A friend I met in the diabetic antenatal clinic had severe problems with sickness however which made control very difficult – at one point the biggest battle was keeping food in her stomach long enough for some carbohydrate to be absorbed and she took to giving her injections after meals for a short time to avoid continual hypos.

At 9 weeks I had a small amount of bleeding one evening and called the GP in. He advised me to go to bed and stay there until it stopped. There were no signs the next morning so I got up in the afternoon to go to my antenatal appointment. Luckily, an ultrasound scan confirmed all was well and also gave me the opportunity to see the baby's heart beating (it looked like a pulsating monkey nut at this point). Apparently this type of occurrence is fairly normal, although it should never be ignored. A surprisingly high proportion of pregnancies end in miscarriage before 12 weeks and medical attention must be sought immediately if you suspect anything is wrong at all. (This fact also makes it sensible not to broadcast news of the impending event too widely until you are over three months).

Things progressed fairly happily for the next few weeks – my HbA$_1$s were coming back at around 7–7.5 and the obstetrician was happy with my rate of weight gain and growth. However in August I hit the next problem. I started having severe hypos with little or no warning symptoms. Throughout my diabetic history I had always had excellent warning of a hypo, never passed out or needed anyone else to bring me round and had always woken should I go hypo in the night. Suddenly I had lost all my warning symptoms entirely and was sinking into deep hypo extremely quickly. One night after struggling to get Lucozade and Hypostop into me for over twenty minutes Kevin was on the verge of reaching for the glucagon when I came round sufficient to slip away from him, out of bed, into the bathroom and lock the door to keep him out. He only just managed to persuade me to come out before he broke the door down! Luckily I had someone with me every time it happened but I began to worry seriously about driving or going out alone, and a few nights away from home at a conference had my colleagues boning up on the use of hypostop and glucagon and knocking on my door if I wasn't seen for longer than a couple of hours.

Hypos are not dangerous for the foetus – research seems to show no ill effect at all – but they obviously carry their own inherent dangers, and also the disruptive effect on control is worrying. The particularly aggressive approach to control during pregnancy can often result in the type of problems I was experiencing and after a HbA$_1$ result of 5.4%, I was advised to ease up a little and reduce my dosages – aiming for average test results of c. 8 mmol rather than c. 6 mmol. This seemed to do the trick and life returned to something more like normal.

At this point I was 4 months gone and had started to look noticeably fatter. At 15 weeks I had had a scan to confirm the dates, and at 18 weeks they took blood to test for the likelihood of foetal abnormality such as Downs Syndrome or spina bifida. This test (AFP test) is not conclusive but can indicate whether further, more invasive and therefore riskier, investigation such as amniocentesis might be recommended. The test came back normal and a further, more detailed scan at 20 weeks showed no apparent abnormalities. This gave relief for a very stressful period for me – by 20 weeks when I was given the all clear I had already started to feel the baby move and was emotionally and mentally already very committed to the pregnancy – if anything abnormal had shown up I really don't know what we would have decided – despite our pre-pregnancy discussions and certainty on such a possibility.

One word about scans – encourage the baby's father to come along – they're amazing! At 15 weeks I could already see all the bones in the fingers and toes – a delight Kevin missed as although he was present for the scan at 20 weeks the baby turned its back on us and refused to co-operate with a 'good picture'.

By October I was in maternity clothes, feeling big and getting bigger! My control was still good – it's amazing how much motivation being pregnant gives you. As the foetus grew, however, so did my insulin needs and throughout October, November and December my dosages were edging up continually. In early December a morning dose of Protaphane was introduced to smooth out early evening and bedtime blood sugars.

Pregnancy is divided into three 'trimesters' – three periods of c. three months. During the middle months of pregnancy the foetus grows steadily, though reasonably slowly, having developed most of its major organs during the first three months. As you enter the third trimester, however, fat begins to be laid down under the skin and the rate of growth increases. At this point diabetic control again becomes crucial, as high blood sugars will lead to an abnormally high rate of growth in the foetus and eventually to a big baby with increased amounts of fat laid down – what is sometimes referred to as a 'diabetic cherub'.

It is this process which leads to many diabetic women having caesarean delivery or early induced birth – if you go all the way to 'term' (i.e. the full forty weeks of pregnancy) the baby can simply grow too big, with obvious problems during birth and also resulting problems for the baby in the first few weeks.

The aim is therefore to achieve blood sugar control as close to that of non-diabetics as possible to ensure that the foetus grows at normal rate. Things were going well for me – I had a scan at 26 weeks (mid November) which showed the baby was exactly on the 'average' line on the graph and the obstetrician had agreed to let me go to term if no problems arose, planning to scan again at 34 weeks. However, in mid-December I caught one of the flu viruses that were doing the rounds and felt terrible for two weeks. I was still working at this point and was extremely tired and run-down. No sooner had I recovered (just in time for Christmas) than I finished work, relaxed, and caught another one over New Year.

In total, there was a period of about 5 weeks when my control slipped distinctly, with my first HbA$_1$s over the 'normal' level. I had real trouble keeping my sugars below 9 mmol and was getting occasional results as high as 15 mmol. I seemed to be continually pumping more and more insulin in with little impact on my sugars and the diabetes team became concerned about insulin resistance, when you have so much insulin drifting round the system that the body simply starts to ignore it. Eventually, I recovered from the flu and my control returned to normal – however the last few weeks had already had their impact.

At 36 weeks gestation, I was feeling pretty good. I was well rested, now being on maternity leave, and although I felt huge I was also quite active, and the end was in sight. Any time I didn't spent in a medical waiting room was taken up with decorating the baby's room (with much help from the two sets of grandparents shopping for the baby and for my hospital stay, making lists(!) and meeting up with other expectant mothers for aqua-natal classes and coffee!

Another daily task was completing my 'kick-chart'. This is a simple system for monitoring the baby's general wellbeing by noting the time each day when you feel the tenth kick or movement. You are advised that if you do not feel ten movements before 6 pm, or if the normal pattern changes drastically, then to contact the hospital. At 33 weeks I had a day when the baby hardly moved all day, and amidst all the obvious fears went to hospital in the evening to be monitored. When you haven't felt anything all day there is nothing as reassuring as the loud thup-thup of the baby's heart trace from the monitor. the next day the baby seemed to be turning somersaults, just to make up!

Earlier in the pregnancy we had decided that we would attend ante-natal classes run by the NCT (National Childbirth Trust. This was definitely an excellent move. The classes themselves were extremely good and thorough, dealing with the emotional and physiological aspects of birth, our rights and expectations from the medical system, different approaches to pain relief and birth, relaxation and assertiveness skills, breastfeeding techniques and infant and child care. These sessions really helped take the fear out of labour and birth, and in themselves were an opportunity to prepare both physically and emotionally for the huge life change about to come – a weekly space for us to concentrate on our baby together. However, they also had a very important social role for both of us, giving Kevin an opportunity to meet and talk to other men also about to become fathers, and for me to swop pregnancy experiences and establish a network of friends for me, and my baby, which has been invaluable.

In week 37, one of the women from the NCT classes had her baby, three weeks early. Suddenly it all started to become frighteningly real.

At nearly 38 weeks, I had a scan which indicated that the baby had continued growing at a rate parallel to the previous scan four weeks earlier – it was still a big baby but, importantly, it hadn't accelerated its growth pattern. I'd worked hard on my diabetic control since the last scan and had been rewarded with almost constant levels of 4.5 mmol. The doctor decided he was happy to leave me a further week, but that I could then expect to be admitted for induction and should come to clinic with my bags in the car.

At this visit I also had a further session on the monitor, as the baby's movements had reduced again, and a very detailed scan, called a BPP, to check the baby's general state of health. This looks at movements (both sudden and general), heart rate, amount of amniotic fluid (in diabetic women there's a tendency for increased amounts and 'respiratory move-ments' (small movements of the chest muscles which look like breathing movements). Each of these five categories are marked out of two giving a total score out of ten. At this point my baby scored eight, as they couldn't see any of the respiratory movements, so a further BPP was booked for the following Monday.

Also at this clinic visit I had a long chat with one of the midwives, Jacky, about what I could expect at the birth. I'd already done a fair bit of research and preparation for the type of birth I wanted and the difficulties I might expect in achieving this. Normally a diabetic woman will have an in-ternal examination at about 38 weeks to assess the chances of induction being successful. If her cervix is still hard and tight, then a caesarian may be offered. If, however, her cer-vix is reasonably 'ripe' (soft and stretchy) and the baby is presenting head down and engaged in the pelvis, then in-duction will be attempted. Initially, pessaries will be inserted which contain a hormone called prostoglandin. This softens the cervix and encourages it to efface (stretch out) and begin to dilate (open). Prostoglandins are also present in seminal fluid, which is one of the reasons why sex is a good way to bring on labour.

The need to deliver a diabetic woman this early in preg-nancy is related to the high risk factor in the last weeks. Ba-bies of diabetic women can grow very large in the last few weeks due to excess fat being laid down and, obviously, if the baby grows too big, delivery will be extremely difficult and a caesarian necessary. However, there is also a risk at-tached to diabetic pregnancies of sudden unexplained still-birth in the final two weeks. Both of these problems are thought to be related to diabetic control, but there has not yet been sufficient cases where control has been excellent throughout pregnancy to be sure that the risk of stillbirth is then concurrent with the non-diabetic population. Under-standably, most obstetricians prefer not to take the gamble.

The other complicating factor is, of course, diabetic control during labour. Labour is one of the most exhausting things you are ever likely to do, putting a huge strain on the body's energy supplies. Even non-diabetic women are tested during labour for the presence of ketones in their urine as the body breaks down fat to meet the overwhelming demand for energy. For diabetic women the danger of hypoglycaemia is obvious, however if blood sugars run too high during labour this increases the risk of ketosis and also has a detrimental effect on the baby after delivery (see later). Added to all this is the fact that women are usually denied any food or drink during labour in hospital in case a general anaesthetic is necessary. Diabetic women are usually controlled with a glucose/insulin drip which is under the control of the midwife and adjusted according to regular blood tests.

A diabetic woman might therefore reasonably expect a very high tech labour, with several drips and wires attached, a high degree of drug controlled pain relief and a low degree of mobility and personal control of the experience. Throughout the pregnancy the prospect of this type of labour had depressed me and I had experienced my first real anger at my diabetes. If I hadn't had diabetes I may well have been requesting a water birth at home, and I was very distressed at what appeared to be a complete lack of choice in the matter of how the birth of my baby should be managed .

On the Thursday I packed my bags into the boot of the car and went to clinic – expecting to be admitted ready for induction the following morning. At this point I was one day off 39 weeks. However, my consultant was happy with the previous week's scan, the BPP results and my general state of health and decided that he would leave me a little longer and admit me the following Wednesday instead – almost another week and only a couple of days off term! This was excellent news, as although he'd agreed several weeks earlier to let me go as close to term as possible, I'd fully expected him to impose the cut-off point at 39 weeks maximum. However the best news was yet to come.

Firstly, prompted by Jacky, the consultant had a long chat to me about the birth and agreed to only intermittent foetal monitoring, to hold back from use of ARM and oxytocin for as long as possible and that I should be allowed to be as mobile as possible throughout. Potentially I had now shed all drips and wires, except the glucose/insulin. This he felt was not up to him, but a matter for my diabetes consultant, although, obstetrically, he was happy for me to look into controlling my own blood sugars.

Secondly, I discovered that even if you are to come into hospital for the birth you can request any midwife you like for labour (providing she agrees) and don't have to simply have whoever is assigned to you from the delivery ward when you arrive (who you have probably never met before). Over my ante-natal visits I had got to know Jacky very well, she knew my feelings as regards the birth, and she had also been doing a lot of extra reading up on diabetic pregnancies and birth. She agreed to attend the birth of our baby.

The next day I rang my diabetes consultant who agreed to let me attempt labour without the glucose/insulin drip. He worked out a regime for me of hourly blood tests, with glucose every hour and fast-acting insulin every four hours. He also gave advice as to how to adjust things if my sugars started rising or falling. I typed up all his advice and stapled it to my birth plan so the information was readily available for anyone involved in my labour. Now I had permission to attempt a totally natural, non-interventionist birth – I couldn't have had any better news!

The following Sunday, at about 3 pm, I had a 'show'. This is when the plug of mucous comes away from the cervix and is discharged, and is a sign that something is starting to happen. At 9.30 pm, with contractions every 3 minutes, we left for the hospital.

When we arrived at hospital I was attached to the monitor for 20 minutes to confirm I was in established labour and assess the condition of the baby. An internal examination found my cervix to be 3–4 cms dilated (you have to be 10 cms dilated before the baby can be born) and Jacky was called to come and look after me. She called my diabetic consultant at c. 1 am to let him know I was in labour and he asked to be rung every four hours in order to check all was OK.

For the next few hours things went really well. I was coping with the pain with just my TENS machine, breathing and relaxation (the NCT classes really came into their own, and I was progressing well, being 8 cms dilated by 3 am. My blood sugars were constantly around 5 mmol – we increased my glucose intake whenever it dropped much below this – and I had no presence of ketones. I was up and about for much of this time, and found being upright and active really helped. We took the mattress off the bed and put in on the floor with plenty of cushions so I could labour, and push, on all fours. Kevin was wonderful; taking responsibility for my blood tests, giving me lots of encouragement and letting me hang on to his hand for hours; and the baby was doing fine both during and between contractions.

However, at c. 5 am I got stuck. I was almost fully dilated, but the contractions were beginnning to slow down and get less effective. My waters still hadn't broken, so Jacky ruptured them at this point in the hope that the pressure of the baby's head would start things up again. It didn't work. At c. 7 am an obstetrician was called who eventually recommended an oxytocin drip. This made my contractions stronger and more regular again, but I managed to remain relaxed and in control, and coped without any drugs.

At about 8.30 am I began to feel the urge to push, and did so with all my strength, for some time. However, despite all our efforts, the baby simply wouldn't come. I was beginning to get extremely tired. At c. 12.30 pm the obstetrician decided to attempt a forceps delivery (i.e. to pull the baby out with forceps) but said he would like to do so in theatre in case it didn't work. In that eventuality they would then be able to go ahead with a caesarian straight away. I was too exhausted to carry on, so we agreed. Kevin was supplied with a theatre gown and mask and I was rushed down the corridor like something out of 'Casualty'.

The forceps didn't work so I was then put under a general anaesthetic for an emergency caesarian section. Hannah was born at 12.58 pm on Monday, 7th February 1994, and weighed in at exactly 11 (yes, eleven) pounds. Her size surprised everyone, including the consultant. General opinion had been that I was likely to have a baby of around 9 lbs, and the fact that she was so big explained why I couldn't push her out.

It is not clear why Hannah was so big – it is easy to blame

diabetes for everything which happens medically and large babies are thought to be related to diabetic control. However my control was consistently good throughout the last few weeks, which is when she must have gained the excess weight, so other factors must also have played a part – maybe I was always destined to have big babies!

I was disappointed not to have given birth, however I did feel I'd given it a good shot. My diabetic control was excellent throughout labour without the glucose/insulin drip, and the active approach to labour, made possible by not being tied down by drips and monitors, definitely enabled me to cope with the pain in a positive way.

Hannah was a very strong baby. Despite my exhaustion, she did not get distressed at all during the labour and birth. She was handed to Kevin a few minutes after being born and he held her until I came round from the anaesthetic 25 minutes later. When I woke up the first thing I saw was my baby and I was able to breastfeed her immediately.

However, after about 5 hours, her blood sugars started to drop and she became hypoglycaemic. This often happens in babies of diabetic mothers and does not mean that the baby is diabetic themselves. Before birth, they become used to the higher than normal sugar level of the mother and produced increased levels of insulin themselves. After birth it can take 2–3 days for their system to stabilise, and as they are not taking in much carbohydrate in their feeds, they become hypo. This can be dangerous for newborns if not treated, and is almost certainly unpleasant! Hannah was taken up to Special Care at 6.30 pm, where she was fed through a naso-gastric tube to ensure she took sufficient carbohydrate. I was still pretty groggy from the operation, and needed to sleep, but it was still very strange not having her with me that first night.

The following day I was able to get as far as a wheelchair (albeit very carefully) and was taken up to see her in Special Care, where I also breastfed her. She fed so well she was able to come back to me 2 hours later and remained with me from then on. We had a minor scare on the third day when her BMs dropped again. My milk hadn't come in yet and she was so jaundiced that she was falling asleep at every feed instead of sucking. I had to give her supplementary bottles of formula for a few hours to keep her sugars up, but she stabilised the next day and the bottles didn't disrupt our establishing breastfeeding, as I'd feared.

Post-natally I was fine, apart from being rather anaemic. My insulin needs had increased by about 300% during pregnancy and I was able to reduce to pre-pregnancy dosages immediately afrer the birth. The caesarian wasn't as bad as it can sound. I was very sore for a few days, but regular pain relieving drugs took care of that. The midwives had me out of bed within hours of the operation and positively encouraged me to get up and about as soon as I felt able. By the third day I was able to look after Hannah completely myself. I had the staples (rather than stitches) out on day 5, and when we went home a week after the birth, I had run up and down the stairs several times before I remembered I had just had a major operation!

Life with a small baby is hard, but very rewarding. As diabetic parents there are simply even more things to complicate matters. The baby always seems to wake and want feeding just as your meal is ready and I forgot my injection more than once in the early days. Also if you are breastfeeding the baby takes a large amount of your calories and carbohydrates, so at the moment I'm eating a huge amount to keep both her and myself fuelled. I'm also ashamed to say that I'm so busy my blood testing regime has returned to nearly its pre-pregnancy disgrace!

Hannah was a week old before she had a name. We eventually settled on Hannah Beth Allen, and only after it was decided did we realise what her initials would be. So, we now have our very own little HbA_1.

I hope this account has been useful, interesting or both! Advice if you are pregnant or thinking about it . . . read everything you can lay your hands on! If you are informed and you understand what is happening to your body it is much easier to do what's best for you and the baby. Also, if you want a less medically managed birth, you are much more likely to get agreement if you have been very well-controlled throughout pregnancy and if you can demonstrate that you understand what might happen and the need to be flexible. Finally, don't worry too much if you are not able to have the type of birth you would ideally want. If it has to be a caesarian, or a heavily managed induced labour, then find out enough to make the most of it in whatever way suits you, and if it doesn't go according to plan? – believe me, the most important thing at the end of the day is the safe delivery of your baby.

LET'S LOOK AT THE ODDS

– if the father has IDDM (Insulin Dependent Diabetes Mellitus), 1 in 20 of his children will develop some form of diabetes
– if the mother has IDDM, 1 in 50 of her children will develop some form of diabetes.
– interestingly, research states that IDDM is passed on more by fathers with IDDM than mothers with IDDM. The risk of the child getting diabetes by the age of twenty is 1.3% if the mother has diabetes compared to 6.1% if the father has diabetes.
– if both parents have IDDM, 1 in 70 of their children will develop some form of diabetes
– 5 to 6% of children with a parent that has IDDM can develop the tendency to get diabetes
– congenital birth defects (heart, kidney defects) are twice as common in diabetic mothers than in non-diabetics – this is thought to be in direct relation to high blood sugars. Once good blood sugar control is achieved this risk is equal to that of non-diabetic mothers.
– a diabetic woman has a 97% chance of having a healthy baby if her diabetes is well controlled, the same as a non-diabetic mother
– your risks are increased with the length of time you've had diabetes and if you have developed any serious complications
– there used to be a lot of talk about diabetics having large babies (over 10 lbs) at birth, this is usually due to excess sugar that has been in the blood. We now know that tighter blood sugar control can help prevent this (unless, of course, your

husband, like mine, is 19 stone, 6 ft. 8 in tall and you are 5 ft. 7in tall, (as I am) and weigh considerably less (as I do!).

Recent evidence shows that your chances of having a healthy baby are greatly increased by maintaining good blood sugar control approximately three months prior to conception and throughout pregnancy. It is especially important during the first six to seven weeks of pregnancy as this is when the babies organs are forming. You can improve these chances if you follow the guidelines.

The key factors are:

CONTROL: good blood sugar control before conception and during pregnancy

COMMITMENT: from you

SUPPORT: from your partner

TEAMWORK: between you and your health care team

THE MENSTRUAL CYCLE

The menstrual cycle affects everyone differently, with diabetetes or not.

As far as having diabetes is concerned, insulin requirements change in approximately 40% of women. Some women increase their insulin dose by up to 20% and others need to decrease it by 10%. The hormones that affect the menstrual cycle also affect the action of insulin.

75% of women with diabetes don't notice a change in their blood sugar levels in relation to their menstrual cycle. Some go hypo two days before and then experience high blood sugars once their cycle starts. With time you'll be able to make adjustments accordingly if you are regular and able to predict when your menstrual cycle is due. If you are not able to predict, you can make adjustments once you start your cycle.

CANDIDIASIS: (thrush)

Women with diabetes are more susceptible to these problems, especially when your blood sugars are out of control and they remain elevated. This occurs because when you are 'spilling' excess sugar, the urine sugar encourages the growth of thrush (a fungus).

The symptoms of thrush are pain and a burning sensation while urinating, swelling and itching. This can all be treated with creams e.g. Canesten, pessaries and tighter blood sugar control.

FERTILITY

Women whose blood sugar control is very poor may have reduced fertility. However if your control is good, fertility is not significantly less than in non-diabetic women. Therefore if pregnancy is not desired, contraception is ESSENTIAL.

SEXUALITY

In researching for this book I found very little information on female sexuality, sexual dysfunction and diabetes. Most of the research is on men. Sexual response is easier to measure with men than with women, it is more obvious, perhaps this is why male sex problems are given more attention.

The majority of women's sexual problems are related to poor diabetes control. Excessive high blood sugars can leave you feeling tired, constantly thirsty and drinking and then constantly going to the loo. This is enough to dampen anybody's sex drive. Once you've sorted out your blood sugars, your libido will more than likely perk up.

The most common complaint and documented subject was the decrease in lubrication during intercourse. This condition can be caused by high blood sugars.

If neuropathy is present, the nerve fibres that stimulate the genitalia may be affected and not able to release the natural lubricating fluids. The use of water soluble lubricants such as KY Jelly are recommended for this condition.

9

Disorderly Eating

EATING DISORDERS
Anorexia/ bulimia/ binging/ dangerous dieting habits +
diabetes = deadly combinations.

Eating disorders are apparently more common in individuals with diabetes than in the general public and those whose diabetes is poorly controlled are at greater risk. The reason for eating disorders are many and varied. There are different reasons for everyone, so each person has to discover the source of their problem. Studies show that eating disorders are associated with efforts to diet. With having diabetes we are predisposed to eating disorders because of the high focus on food and the need for 'control'. It's easy to become obsessed as we need to plan everything. If we're going out for the day we must consider if we need to pack a lunch or bring along extra fruit. We think of where our next meal will be, what type of food we will have and most importantly, when will we have it. Talk about STRESS!

This eating pattern can make us more susceptible especially when hypos are involved. There's a catch 22 with hypos – overeating for fear of them and overeating because of them. A fear of hypos encourages eating. It's easier to eat more rather than to eat less for fear of having a hypo later. Then, when we have hypos we often over-treat them, end up eating far too much (usually something too sweet, with no nutritional value and fattening) and this can leave us feeling terribly guilty and depressed because it goes against everything that we are taught about good diabetes control.

Excessive compulsive ways to lose weight are all harmful to our health. This includes using laxatives, self-induced vomiting, obsessive exercising, binging and purging, deliberately reducing or eliminating your insulin, fasting, fad diets.

In young women, lack of nourishment can cause physical damage and lead to poor physical development.

That's why it's necessary to balance a healthy diet, insulin regime, and exercise programme for proper growth development.

Individuals with diabetes who have eating disorders and poorly controlled blood sugars are at a greater risk of developing more serious complications and at an earlier age than those who manage a healthier lifestyle.

'PEOPLE WITH EATING DISORDERS VALUE THEMSELVES ACCORDING TO THEIR SIZE AND SHAPE and sometimes need help to see their true value as a unique individual.'

TREATMENT FOR EVERYONE

The first step to treatment is identifying and acknowledging the problem. If you're not ready to talk to a doctor or nurse or anyone about your eating problem, maybe you can start to look into it yourself.

1 – Get yourself a diary. Take it with you everywhere and RECORD EVERYTHING (including the good, the bad, and the ugly).

RECORD:

– time of day
– your emotions, how you feel mentally
– how you feel physically
– what you've eaten
– what you've drunk
– blood glucose results
– insulin dose
– if you've vomited
– what you were doing at the time before you binged, what triggered it off (was it an emotion or an event)

2 – With this recorded information can you see any sort of

pattern? See if you can recognise what triggers it off.

3 – Once you have some insight into this you might be more prepared to discuss it.

Below I've listed the symptoms of various eating disorders. If you fall under any of these categories you'll know what you're working against. There are a number of self-help books written on this topic which you can read. If this is too difficult and you want to TALK to someone about it, you can seek guidance from a professional. If you can, get expert help and find one that has an interest in diabetes (through your G.P., consultant, diabetes nurse specialist or the British Eating Disorders Assoc.) They know how to help as they are specifically trained for this. Remember that they also WANT to help, this is why they are involved in this line of care. At first it might be difficult because with having diabetes and an eating disorder you have double the guilt of not following a diet/meal plan as you should. This can make it twice as hard for you to talk about it. Just remember, be honest with someone about your eating disorder instead of pretending that your diabetes is in poor control for some unexplained reason.

You can seek help on a one to one basis or get involved in group therapy meetings. This is often very successful as you will be meeting people with similar problems. You will see for yourself that you are normal and not alone in this situation. Everyone in this group is there to help each other.

It's important to get help as soon as possible. The longer you wait, the more damage you are causing to your body and the more difficult it will be to overcome it. Also, it will come as a relief to get it out into the open and know that YOU are trying to do something about it.

Take it one step at a time and one day at a time.

The first thing to realise is that you are not alone. Many people suffer from the same experiences and difficulties.

WITH THE PROPER HELP YOU CAN OVERCOME THIS

Remember, like all other areas of your health, it's crucial that you shop around until you find a therapist you feel happy with.

BINGES

I am by all means not your 'perfect little diabetic'. I can honestly say that I've had my share of Mars Bar binges. I think it's perfectly normal and natural behaviour! I also think it's normal behaviour to crave or want to eat some of the 'forbidden' foods and over-indulge. EVERYONE does it, every now and again.

There's no way that you should feel guilty for going off your 'diet'. How many people do you know who have stuck to a diet for 10 years? (or for however long you've had diabetes). As long as it's a once-in-a-while indulgence and you keep your blood sugar in check, you'll be alright, and probably happier for it.

It's when you get past the odd binge and make a habit of it that there should be cause for concern.

Anorexia and bulimia have many features in common. Some individuals have both and some go from one to the other, often it's from bulimia to anorexia.

ANOREXIA NERVOSA

Anorexia is defined as the lack of desire for food. Anorexia Nervosa is a serious psychological condition and is more common in young women than the rest of the population. The most startling thing about people with anorexia is the way they see themselves. They are very underweight yet see themselves as being grossly overweight.They are obsessed with food yet they eat very little. They're afraid of gaining any weight and an extra pound or two can leave them feeling withdrawn and depressed. They often have a low self esteem and lack of confidence and will deny they have a problem even when it is painstakingly obvious to others.

A personality trait of an anorexic is someone who is a perfectionist. As slimness and self-control are highly valued in our society, we can see the attraction to anorexia nervosa, particularly with young, vulnerable women.

The main symptom is the relentless pursuit of thinness through self starvation and a fear of becoming fat.

Symptoms often include:

- severe weight loss
- distortion & misconceptions about weight and body size/shape
- excessive exercising
- vomiting/purging
- isolation – loss of friends
- emotional irritable behaviour
- difficulty in sleeping
- loss of menstrual periods
- perfectionism
- feeling cold, poor circulation
- growth of downy hair all over body

BULIMIA NERVOSA:

Characterised by binge eating followed by self induced vomiting, periods of starvation and/or purging with laxatives; sufferers often move to bulimia from anorexia.
Symptoms often include:

- binge eating large amounts of food
- vomiting and/or purging
- often disappearing to the lavatory after meals in order to get rid of food eaten
- secretive behaviour
- feeling out of control, helpless and lonely
- menstrual disturbances
- sore throat and erosion of tooth enamel caused by vomiting
- dehydration, poor skin condition
- lethargy
- emotional behaviour and mood swings
- devious and deceptive behaviour

Reproduced by permission from the British Eating Disorder Association.

THE EATING DISORDERS ASSOCIATION

EDA is a self help organisation which aims to help everyone who is involved with bulimia or anorexia nervosa by:

– Supporting sufferers and their families and friends
– Providing information
– Developing new thinking and understanding about eating disorders.

See appendix for address.

10

Body Image

A few years ago I worked as a professional model. This profession, made me understand what body image is all about. Trying to fit diabetes into this life-style often proved to be a challenge.

The worst situations were having a hypo just before a photo shoot. It wouldn't have been so bad had I not been modelling bathing suits. I tended to over-treat my hypos in those days and as a result, this would leave me feeling stuffed, bloated and as fat as a rhino.

Believe me when I say it wasn't exactly easy to portray the sylph, vixen, beach bunny I was made up to look like. To make matters worse, I'd then have the make-up artist in hysterics because I'd be wiping the chocolate off my mouth and perspiration from my face after she'd just spent 1 hour applying my professional layer of make-up.

The beauty business is a massive industry which sells false hopes and fantasy. They want to persuade women into thinking that if we buy their products, we will look like the models in their advertisements. They want us to think that if we use these products, we will also be ravishing, desirable, youthful and beautiful.

Many of these advertisements use models that are 13 to 16 years old who are actually made up to look years older. Brooke Shields started posing in her Calvin Kleins at the ripe old age of 13 and became an instant success and favourite for advertisers worldwide.

There is an enormous amount of pressure for women to conform to skinny stereotypes seen in advertising. With perfect looking models in fashion magazines in newstands everywhere; in television commercials and on billboards. We're SURROUNDED with these images. It's hard not to feel that we have to live up to them and get discouraged when we can't (and shouldn't) live up to these unrealistic images. How many times have you said to yourself 'If only I could lose 10 lbs... I'd get that perfect job or partner (or both!)'. There's something about being a woman in today's society that can easily lead us to a distorted body image.

In modelling, the female body version is not normal. Today, models in general are 4–5 inches taller and weigh 23% less than the average woman, a generation ago they weighed about 8% less than the average. With these waif-like images around it is not difficult to see why so many normal women think they are fat and imperfect. We're being fooled into thinking we're overweight and out of shape. Society places enormous pressure on us to want to do just about anything in order to have the same lithe and lissom body of today's Super Models, regardless of our natural shape or bone structure. The fight to sell products whether it's for clothing, make-up or memberships to health spas is an enormously profitable business. The diet industry alone is a £16 billion-a-year industry. So advertisers are not about to let up and let us think that we're alright.

We often use the mannequins in the ads as role models, we want to emulate them. The ad tells us that if we buy the garment that's modelled, then we can look like or as good as the model wearing it. This can lead to a distorted body image as more often than not, the opposite is true. No matter how slim or fit you are, you'll think or see yourself as not looking good enough.

Little do most people know that these 'perfect' images on celluloid are painstakingly created with special effects. The cover photograph on a magazine is often air-brushed to conceal any imperfections on the model such as: blemishes, wrinkles, moles (except Cindy Crawford's of course), scars and so on. Other techniques used are special lighting, make-up, poses and camera angles.

So the next time you look at a magazine cover, don't get depressed thinking you could never look as attractive as the model, remember the 'tricks of the trade' and think of how awesome you would look in a photo if the same techniques were used.

The ideals of beauty are forever changing. Jean Shrimpton (pencil thin) was all the rage in the 60s, Cheryl Tiggs (fresh, slim, all-American) in the 70s, Elle MacPherson (chesty, muscular, lean) in the 80s and from Claudia Schiffer and Cindy Crawford (both are very voluptous) to Kate Moss (the Super Waif) in the 90s. You can notice the changes, and the advertising world is just starting to get a bit more realistic with the images they are using, but they still have a long way to go before they resemble what the average female form really looks like. Though I don't think that will ever happen because we all want to dream and all want to achieve the unattainable.

So, if you're thinking of getting breast implants this year, save your money. Next year a flat chest and no hips will probably be all the rage. Women of all shapes and sizes can be and look beautiful, healthy, glamorous, sexy and desirable.

People often compare themselves to their friends or people they see on the street and not taking into consideration that everyone has different bone structures. A lot of the way we look has to do with heredity. We're the product of our genes. Body weight is as genetically determined as our own height.

You can lose or gain weight to suit your height but there is very little you can do about bone structure. Cosmetic surgery is a desperate costly alternative. Several well known actresses, who already had beautiful figures, have had ribs removed to appear slimmer and more attractive with an hour glass figure. The hollywood stars really aren't the 'perfect' women they're meant to portray. In the movie 'Pretty Woman' a skinnier look-alike (a body double) was used to replace Julia Roberts in the love scenes with Richard Gere.

What is encouraging is that you can make the best of what nature gave you – by eating a healthy diet and exercising, whether it's by toning up, lifting weights, or doing aerobics. Be realistic as you can only change so much.

You'll feel great knowing that you've accomplished something for yourself and that you look as good as YOU can. You'll be healthier in body and mind by doing this. Just compare how you feel after a 2 hour cycle ride to how you feel after watching television for 2 hours.

You'll have your good days as well as your bad days. It

will not only make you look better, you'll feel better about yourself and the real bonus is your blood sugar control will be easier to achieve and maintain. Set yourself reasonable goals and JUST GO FOR IT!

47% OF BRITISH WOMEN ARE SIZE 16 OR OVER

'Women see pictures of us and wonder, 'Why don't I look like that?' What they don't realise is, WE don't even look like that.'

Stephanie Seymour,
Supermodel

Men also have pressure on them, though I don't believe it's to the same degree as women. Men have the images of Mel Gibson, Arnold Schwartzeneggar and the Chippendales to contend with or live up to.

But I really think women, more than men, place more importance on how they look, often their entire self worth depends on how they look. How many times have you heard a guy say 'If only I could lose 10 lbs before the office Christmas party!'. Also, men rarely complain of having their 'fat days and their skinny days'. Unfortunately it's society's fault that women are valued more for how they look than for their personalities or for what they do.

The bottom line is : you can MAKE THE BEST OF WHAT YOU'VE GOT!

Take a positive step and try and focus on the parts of yourself that you do like by highlighting and emphasising them.

11

Miscellaneous

WEIGHT GAIN AFTER DIAGNOSIS

It is expected and perfectly normal to gain weight after diagnosis and commencement of insulin treatment. More than likely you lost a considerable amount of weight before diagnosis and found that you rapidly put it on after.

This can be quite discouraging, especially if you are doing everything to achieve proper blood sugar control. This weight gain is caused by rehydration. Before diagnosis you were dehydrated therefore your weight gain after diagnosis is mainly water. The struggle to maintain the weight pre-diagnosis can be the trigger to an eating disorder. Be prepared and learn how to stabilise your weight once you establish a routine.

Excessive weight gain can also be caused by too much insulin which then causes cravings and eating to balance the insulin. Another problem can be caused by blood sugars dropping to 'hypo' level during the night without knowing it; the body then corrects the blood sugar and results in a high blood glucose in the morning. The cure for this is less insulin at night, but you may be tempted to increase the insulin because of the high morning blood glucose. Bingo ... you're now eating to balance the insulin > a vicious circle. The medical profession is beginning to realise that this happens alot and may be one of the things that precipitates eating disorders.

THE UNDERUSE AND MISUSE OF INSULIN

It's important to talk about this subject at the risk of instructing people on how to induce glycosuria (the presence of large amounts of sugar in the urine) a.k.a. 'spilling' sugar.

The misuse of insulin to influence body weight is common in young women with diabetes. Some even go so far as saying 'It's the only good thing about having diabetes!' This happens when an insulin injection is omitted altogether or the person is not giving a sufficient amount of insulin to cover their diet and keep their blood sugars at a controlled level.This causes the blood sugar to rise and 'spill' into the urine and a rapid weight loss follows. This is the same process that happens pre-diagnosis, which is why you lost weight then. This deliberate means of weight reduction is extremely dangerous. It can lead to ketoacidosis which, if goes untreated , can lead to a coma and death. What happens, is that the part of the body's cells that are protein and fat are broken down and reformed as carbohydrates. If you find yourself using this method, talk about it, share it, get it out in the open and ask for help if you can't stop.There's nothing at all wrong with asking for help.

You may not realise the damage you are causing until it is too late. You may accept the possibility of complications thinking that you are invincible, they couldn't possibly happen to you.

Your concern for weight loss is immediate and the complications are long term making it more difficult to see the apparent damage you are causing.

CHEAT!

Being accused of cheating on our diabetes control can lead to some unpleasant situations. It can leave you feeling self conscious because of always having to eat. Some will hide and eat anywhere but in front of others.

No one wants to feel that they are different and if you're a few pounds overweight, you're already self-conscious about eating. You're afraid of what people will think and say and this could lead you to eating in privacy. I for one, used to do it especially when I was in school.

A lot of people hide sweets and eat them 'behind closed

doors'. You might have a sweet tooth and once in a while, like most people, you crave something sweet. But because you have diabetes you are made to feel that you can't indulge openly, therefore you hide it. This takes us to the 'Bathroom Disease Syndrome'. Somehow, devouring a chocolate eclair in the bathroom loses a bit of the pleasure. Often it's the only place to go when you feel that it's just not worth the hassle and grief that you'll get from your family or partner.

When you get tired of these hassles let the other person know how you feel, how it feels to be accused and called a cheat. Remind them that you are only human and once in awhile you will slip because your needs are just as great as anybody else's.

It's important to understand that the removal of all sweets, desserts and carbohydrates is in fact unhealthy. Psychologically it can leave you feeling deprived, it's even more of a temptation because we often want what we can't have, and physically your body requires carbohydrates for energy. With good understanding and education (and some willpower) you should be able to eat and drink in a manner to satisfy your own inner needs and make your friends and family forget about you having diabetes. The occasional indulgence shouldn't cause you to feel too much guilt. The important thing to remember is don't let it get out of hand and become a habit and make sure that overall you still balance your blood sugars.

Also try to remember that the people questioning you are only trying to look out for you and help you. Very often they are misinformed and think that people with diabetes are never allowed sweets and don't know that you can make up for it, e.g. if you're about to participate in sports or even that you simply need it because your blood sugar is too low.

THE BATHROOM DISEASE

I believe diabetics spend more time in loos than anybody else. We often go there to give our needles and test our blood sugar. Some of us even go there to eat 'forbidden foods' (you know what I'm talking about) because we don't want people to comment on what or how much we are eating, especially if you are female.

Well, we really shouldn't be bothered by what others might think or say when we inject or test in public. Even if your sister tells you that the man on the bus sitting beside you is pulling faces. How does he think you feel as the needle is actually going in YOU. It's something that you have to do so why jeopardise your health and well-being because of what you think others might be thinking.

As long as you are discreet about it, there's no problem. And that means if you're at a dinner table and must give your injection, use a site on your thigh or stomach as it'll be below the table top. There's nothing like seeing someone give an injection in their arm before the first course. There's no need to show off, use your common sense. Insulin pens are perfect in these situations as they don't even look like needles and they're so convenient. Just dial your dose and away you go, no need to fuss with vials and syringes and getting air bubbles out, as it can be more difficult to be discreet with that method.

One of the greatest pieces of advice I was ever given by a doctor was 'I don't care if you are meeting with the Queen of England, if you need something to eat and are having a hypo, pull out that banana or whatever you have on you and eat it – there and then!' It takes guts to do this (I'm sure Liz would understand) but I think it's probably less embarrassing to eat or drink in front of someone than to actually have a hypo and get all sweaty and confused.

It might take awhile before you feel comfortable enough to do this, but take your time and eventually you will have the confidence to be able to do it, and then you'll really be looking after NUMBER ONE.

DEALING WITH THE HANDICAP OF THE GENERAL PUBLIC

I've always said, 'Diabetes is the invisible disease'. It has a different social acceptance compared with other chronic illnesses, such as cerebral palsy, because it is not visible. Having diabetes is not obvious, there are no physical signs.

This is why it is difficult for people who are not associated with someone that has diabetes to understand the magnitude of the condition and all that it entails.

Hence the title of this book, 'FUNNY, YOU DON'T LOOK LIKE A DIABETIC!' How many times have you heard this comment after you have just told someone that you have diabetes? The second most popular comment is 'Oh, my Great Auntie Ethel had diabetes and she's blind because of it!'. Or better still 'My Uncle Fred died because of diabetes!'. Most people who don't actually know what to say, aren't too sure of how they should comment. They're uncomfortable and are trying to relate and not meaning to harm.

Before you get frustrated and annoyed with their remarks, just think back to the time before you were diagnosed. How much did you know about diabetes then?

So, you really can't blame them for their ignorance this time. How much do you know about other illnesses like cancer or tuberculosis. Chances are, very little, unless you work in the medical field or have close ties with someone that suffers from these illnesses.

Since the majority of people with diabetes (90%) have Type II diabetes (non-insulin dependent), most peoples limited knowledge of diabetes is through their acquaintance with these individuals. Type II diabetes is very different from Type I.

Type I is controlled by diet, exercise and insulin. At diagnosis the average age is 12 years old and the individual is usually thin. With Type II, it's controlled by pills and or diet/exercise. Diagnosis usually occurs during adulthood and the individual is usually overweight. This explains why most people say to us, 'Oh, that's not too bad, you just have to watch what you eat, don't you?'

This is why it is up to each and every one of us to educate people in our own way. Just tell them the basics, don't overload them with the information you have sponged since diagnosis. The technical details of blood testing and food values will only confuse them. Answer their questions honestly and don't feel embarrassed, afraid or ashamed. Most people care and ask questions because they are curious and want to learn and at the same time you'll be dispelling some of the gazillion myths about diabetes. So the next time someone says 'You can't have any of these cream cakes, can you, poor thing?' you can answer this very common question by saying 'Actually I can eat them but I've already eaten enough for lunch, thank you for the offer though' or state that you can eat pretty much anything as long as you balance your insulin, blood sugars and exercise accordingly.

WORKING WITH/AGAINST THE MEDIA

There are 180,000 charitable organisations registered in England and Wales alone. The competition to raise funds for these charities is fierce.

There are two arguments, one for and one against the advertisements used to solicit funds for diabetes associations. The arguments against the ads are that for the diabetics themselves, particularly the newly diagnosed, they can be very disconcerting.

An advertisement for the BDA states how a girl 'lives under the shadow of diabetes and how people with diabetes are more likely to suffer from blindness, kidney trouble or amputations.' My heart went out to a boy who told me how upset he was after seeing this poster in a tube station soon after he was diagnosed with diabetes.

However, I think there is an even stronger argument for the advertisements they use. With so much competition for charitable donations, advertisers need to revert to shock value, to grab for attention. The object of these advertisements is to make people stop and think and realise just how serious diabetes is. Remember what I said about it being an 'invisible disease'.

There is no point in showing photos of fit, healthy diabetics because our cause wouldn't seem as great, and the donations would go elsewhere instead of towards diabetes research to find a cure. With the economic climate the way it is these days, there are limited corporate dollars for charities. Therefore, they must appear as critical and needy as they can.

The important factor to remember is that people with diabetes do lead healthy and productive lives. Just look at some of the many famous role models we have: Gary Mabbutt (Footballer, Tottenham Hotspur), Elaine Strich (Actress), Steve James (Snooker player), Tony Pigott (Cricketer, Sussex), Colin Dexter (Author of Inspector Morse), Mary Tyler Moore (Actress), Willie Rushton (Comedian), Sue Lloyd (Actress), Lisa Harrow (Actress), Miles Davis (Jazz Musician), Ella Fitzgerald (Singer).

And the famous role models from the past: Ernest Hemingway, Mario Puzo, H. G. Wells, Thomas Edison, Howard Hughes, Spencer Tracy, Elvis Presley, Dizzie Gillespie.

THE OPATHY PROBLEM:
Nephropathy, Retinopathy, Neuropathy

I won't bore you with what the actual 'complications' of diabetes are, as they are well documented. I do however think it's important to mention the following because it is not well documented and to let you know that you're not alone if you have any of these fears.

The inability for doctors to predict who will suffer from complications can leave us feeling helpless, anxious and depressed at times.

You don't have to keep these thoughts to yourself. If you're about to go for some treatment, e.g. laser treatment, it's often a good idea to talk to someone who has been through the same experience. You'll learn what to expect, what the treatment involves and that it is not as scary as you always feared it would be.

Dealing with the agony and fear of complications can leave you feeling insecure and alone. By discussing these feelings with other people, be it another person with diabetes, your doctor, nurse or a family member, you will learn that people will understand and care about you just the same. Also it will feel good because a load will have been lifted from your shoulders.

You might hear stories of diabetics who are blind or have had a limb amputated or other diabetes related complica-

tions –'Freddy Krugar' type stories – but if you educate yourself on this subject you will be able to put everything into
perspective.

Many of the emotional problems associated with complications are because of the lack of knowledge in this area. It
shouldn't be a taboo subject. If you have questions, ask your
doctor/nurse for straight answers – it is your right to know.
Alternatively, you can look up this information in journals
and diabetes magazines. Most of the stories you've heard
about diabetes and complications are probably unfounded
and grossly exaggerated.

A lot of the statistics that you read are from research that
was conducted 10, 15 or even 20 years ago. This was all before the modern methods of treatment that we have today.
Diabetes treatment has changed dramatically over the years.
Technical advances in medicine such as home blood sugar
monitoring and new insulin therapy (multi-injections with
an insulin pen) have allowed for tighter diabetes control, hence
better long term health, as proven by the DCCT results.

Also, we've taken great strides, and will continue to do so,
in the treatment of complications. In most cases, laser treatment can prevent the development of retinopathy and if protein in the urine is detected early, potential kidney damage
can be avoided. (This is all the more reason to have frequent
medical check-ups at your diabetes clinic.)

12

The Health Care Team

The relationship between the health care team and the person with diabetes is a special one. It is unique in that the person with diabetes takes all roles of the team once he/she leaves clinic and it's an ongoing relationship both when you are sick and when you are well. More responsibility is placed on someone who has diabetes than on any other condition.

DIABETES SPECIALIST NURSE: a qualified Nurse Clinician who has extended training in all aspects of diabetes care.

DIETITIAN: provides guidelines and appropriate nutritional advice.

CONSULTANT: overall head of the team and director of medical care.

CHIROPODIST: provides important specialist help for all aspects of foot care.

CLINICAL PSYCHOLOGIST/PSYCHIATRIST: deals in matters of emotional state with counselling; coping skills, adjusting, problem solving.

With their guidance, you become all members of the health care team.

The responsibility of your treatment lies with yourself. The care for diabetes is unique, unlike other chronic illnesses where the doctor administers to all the needs of the patient. With diabetes your are a major part of a health team that works together: you all have the same goals of maintaining good health.

THE WHITE COAT SYNDROME

It's a common reaction to feel intimidated in front of your doctor. It seems that as soon as he/she puts on their white coat you begin to feel awkward, as if you are talking to a superior being and because you don't want to disappoint them you might fudge your blood sugar testing diaries and lie to them about your overall control.

I was guilty of this during my first few years after diagnosis. The night before my clinic appointment I'd fill in my test book with fictitious results. It would soon resemble a perfect picture of a beautiful blue ocean with the odd brown or orange sailboat thrown in for good measure. These were the days before home blood sugar monitoring and we used colour pencils to record our urine test results. Blue represented negative: no sugar and brown or orange meant positive: that you had sugar in your urine. Little did I know, or understand, that when my doctor saw the test results from my HbA_1 he would quickly know that I was not exactly telling the truth.

It's important to remember that doctors are there because they want to help us and they do care about our health. They also feel like failures when we don't take care of our health. Otherwise they wouldn't have committed themselves to 6–8 years of medical school and continued with the long hours and hard work. And with the structure of the NHS, you certainly can't say that they're in it for the money.

Don't ever be afraid to ask questions. You might think that your questions are stupid or that your doctor/nurse has never heard of them before. It's more than likely that they've heard it all before and they are expecting you to ask. If you don't understand something ask and keep asking until you get it. You have the right to participate in decisions concerning your health. Don't forget that they are also there to learn and they can learn from your questions and experiences. There is no shame in feeling vulnerable and asking for help. The situation will only get worse if you keep it to yourself.

DON'T TELL DOCTORS WHAT YOU THINK THEY WANT TO HEAR
(with this attitude, neither of you benefit)

IT'S OK TO TELL DOCTORS THAT YOUR CONTROL HASN'T BEEN GOOD

DOCTOR/PATIENT RELATIONSHIP

The key words here are HONEST and OPEN COMMUNI-CATION.

Lack of compassion from doctors is probably the most common complaint. A good reason for this is that in medical school, there are very few courses that deal with emotions, the main focus is on the clinical aspects of health. Let your doctor know if you need emotional support. If he is not able to give it then he will be able to direct you to another health professional who can.

As you are the one who has to live with diabetes day in and day out, you know your body and what will and will not work with your routines. This is where your doctor must listen and consider what you are saying in order to meet a healthy compromise. Your doctor must look at the whole picture: all of you, and not just the blood sugars. He must be willing to consider your personality, vocation, life-style, and family as all of these factors influence your diabetes control.

The ideal relationship between doctor and patient can be achieved when both parties agree on how to work towards the same goals.

Clinics are often very busy and rushed, so it's a good idea to be prepared before you go in. This way you are getting the most out of your time and the health care teams' time as well.

It's often a good idea to write down any questions you have before you see your doctor as it's easy to forget them once you're in the clinic and get distracted or feel shy/scared. Be organised and you will save time but don't finish until you're satisfied with your answers.

Be open to suggestions to see someone other than your doctor. If you attend a teaching hospital chances are that you'll be seen by a junior doctor instead of your consultant. Diabetes specialist nurses also play a key role in diabetes care, they are often the ones running the clinics, and are the experts in diabetes care.

CHANGING CLINICS OR DOCTORS

If you're not happy or satisfied with your health care treatment, then do something about it! IT'S YOUR HEALTH, TAKE CHARGE. A friend of mine hasn't been to her clinic for over a year because she doesn't get along with her doctor. By doing this, she's only harming HER health, certainly not her doctor's. Frequent visits to your clinic can be very beneficial for many reasons, along with addressing your immediate concerns, your doctor can pick up on any early warning signs of complications. This is of particular importance in the case of retinopathy and nephropathy as early detection can help prevent further damage.

You must be able to work with your health care team. If there are problems try and discuss them with the people involved. If you find this too difficult, write a letter to them and explain the situation. In this instance it's O.K. to be 'pushy', be assertive and don't ever forget that it's YOUR health therefore your right to pursue the care you deserve.

Just because a particular doctor or certain clinic has been 'assigned' to you, it doesn't mean that you're stuck there for life. Not everyone will get along with people they are assigned to. If this is the situation then you can and should do something about it. You'll be doing yourself, and your doctor a favour as well, if neither of you gets along.

If a referral is required before you change consultants, then explain the situation to your GP. Or if it's your GP that you don't get along with, see if your consultant can refer you to another one. This might take some time but stand by your guns, it's your health and it should be your no.1 priority. Your health care is far too important to push aside in the hope that it will improve on its own, because it won't. This is where you're in control, and only you can do something about it.

If you're not sure of how to go about finding a new doctor, consult your local health authority or Community Health Council. Ask friends for recommendations and visit the clinic to check out the atmosphere and see if you're comfortable with it. Remember, you are the consumer. The doctor, though an expert, is someone who is employed to provide a service.

If you're not satisfied, you can take your custom elsewhere. If you are treated under the NHS this might be more difficult to accomplish than if you were treated privately, but it's not to say that it can't be done.

When I first moved to the Oxford region I went to my local health clinic to register with a new GP. There are six GPs working there and I was assigned to one who had a specialist interest in diabetes. I personally prefer to see a consultant for my diabetes care rather than a GP because I feel they are the 'specialist'. So I asked the GP for a referral to see one I had heard of at the hospital. It was just as well as I felt uncomfortable with his attitude and procedures. Needless to say this particular GP was not too impressed with my request. I think he felt he could monitor my treatment quite adequately. I was then given a referral to see the consultant at the hospital. Upon my second meeting with this GP, my negative feelings for him increased so I wrote a letter to another GP I had met within the clinic, on another visit, stating that I would rather be under his care for GP services. There is a simple card you need to fill out (your GP clinic will give you one) and it's not necessary for you to give any reason whatsoever for your decision to change doctors. Because if need be, it is your right to do so! I took the matter into my own hands, I was taking care of my needs as a patient and made sure that the GP I was assigned to was someone that I felt comfortable discussing my health with and knowing he/she was competent to deal with it.

WHAT DIABETES CARE TO EXPECT – BDA STATEMENT

WHEN YOU HAVE JUST BEEN DIAGNOSED, YOU SHOULD HAVE:

– full medical examination;
– a talk with a registered nurse who has a special interest in diabetes. She/he will explain what diabetes is and talk to you about your individual treatment;
– a talk with a state registered dietitian , who will want to know what you are used to eating and will give you basic

advice on what to eat in the future. A follow-up meeting should be arranged for more detailed advice;
– a discussion on the implications of diabetes on your job, driving, insurance, prescription charges etc, and whether you need to inform the DVLA and your insurance company, if you are a driver;
– information about the BDA's services and details of your local BDA group;
– ongoing education about your diabetes and the beneficial effects of exercise, and assessments of your control.

YOU SHOULD BE ABLE TO TAKE A CLOSE FRIEND OR RELATIVE WITH YOU TO EDUCATIONAL SESSIONS IF YOU WISH.

PLUS:

IF YOU ARE TREATED BY INSULIN:

– frequent sessions for basic instruction on injection technique, looking after insulin and syringes, blood glucose and ketone testing and what the results mean;
– supplies of relevant equipment;
– discussion about hypoglycaemia (hypos): when and why it may happen and how to deal with it.

IF YOU ARE TREATED BY TABLETS:

– a discussion about the possibility of hypoglycaemia (hypos) and how to deal with it;
– instruction on blood or urine testing and what the results mean, and supplies of relevant equipment.

IF YOU ARE TREATED BY DIET ALONE:

– instruction on blood or urine testing and what the results mean, and supplies of relevant equipment.

ONCE YOUR DIABETES IS REASONABLY CONTROLLED, YOU SHOULD:

– have access to the diabetes team at regular intervals – annually if necessary. These meetings should give time for discussion as well as assessing diabetes control;
– be able to contact any member of the health care team for specialist advice when you need it;

– have more education sessions as you are ready for them;
– have a formal medical review once a year by a doctor experienced in diabetes.

AT THIS REVIEW:

– your weight should be recorded;
– your urine should be tested for ketones and protein;
– your blood should be tested to measure long term control.
– you should discuss control, including your home monitoring results;
– your blood pressure should be checked;
– your vision should be checked, and the back of the eyes examined. A photo may be taken of the back of your eyes. If necessary you should be referred to an opthalmologist;
– your legs and feet should be examined to check your circulation and nerve supply if necessary you should be referred to a state registered chiropodist;
– your injection sites should be examined if you are on insulin;
– you should have the opportunity to discuss how you are coping at home and at work.

YOUR ROLE:

– you are an important member of the care team so it is essential that you understand your own diabetes to enable you to be in control of your condition;
– you should ensure you receive the prescribed care from your local diabetes clinic, practice or hospital. If these services are not available to you, you should:
– Contact your GP to discuss the daibetes care available in your area
– Contact your local Community Health Council
– Contact the BDA or your local branch

These guidelines were first produced in 1986 and revised in November 1992.

The control of your diabetes is important, and so is the detection and treatment of any complication. Make sure you are getting the medical care and education you need to ensure you stay healthy.

Printed with permission from the British Diabetic Association.

If you feel you are not getting the treatment you deserve from your GP or hospital clinic then you should write a letter to your local Community Health Council (address in your Yellow Pages) and also to the Diabetes Care Department of the B.D.A. and explain your situation.

PART II

Reviewed by
DR DAVID LESLIE
Consultant Physician

13

Introduction to Exercise

Exercise is as important as diet and insulin in the diabetes triad, yet it receives the least amount of attention both from the health care team and the individual with diabetes. Upon diagnosis we are given many diet sheets and insulin charts to follow but it's a rare clinic that gives us exercise programmes and adequate information on this topic to allow us to complete the triad as best we can.

I was never much of a sports buff before I was diagnosed with diabetes; I never made the school basketball or volleyball teams; in fact, I often dreaded P.E. class. It wasn't until I entered college that I really got involved in any sort of competitive sports and this was mainly because I was trying to bury my school nicknames ('BUFFALOBUTT' & 'THUNDERTHIGHS') and improve my fragile ego and image.

So I figured I needed to try an exercise that would improve my 'problem areas'. I then discovered the 10 speed road bike and the cycling team and actually enjoyed it all. I quickly became motivated, shed the excess body clay and was soon able to don a pair of those black lycra cycling shorts. All the exercise I was doing improved my diabetes control, and I never felt better both mentally and physically! Once I noticed and realised the benefits of exercise to diabetes control I began to make it part of my routine.

This section on exercise was written with assistance from experts on diabetes and exercise. It is designed to motivate you: to get you started or to keep you involved with your current fitness programme and to educate you. It will provide guidelines to follow for everyone from the beginner to the seasoned athlete.

14

Motivation

In order to stay with something, one has to remain motivated. The greatest motivating factor to exercise has to be the many ·POSITIVE BENEFITS:

– increase the body's sensitivity to insulin (therefore reducing insulin requirements)
– muscle activity improves the uptake of insulin
– helps lower blood sugar during and after an exercise session
– improves cardiovascular system, muscle tone and nerve 'tone'
– helps you to lose excess weight
– encourages self-discipline
– increases confidence which contributes to a positive healthier attitude on life
– reduces 'stress hormones' (anxiety, depression and hostility): the added benefit for those of us with diabetes is that a reduction in stress has been shown to improve blood sugar control
– increases libido with improved body image
– you'll sleep better
– long term benefit: a positive outcome down the road

MAXIMISE THE BENEFITS
MINIMISE THE RISKS

Regular exercise can help to minimise the long term effects of having diabetes. A person in good physical shape can better tolerate the physiological stress caused by diabetes. So by staying fit you can counter-act some of the negatives!

All of this will make diabetes more manageable and give

you more time and energy to concentrate on the more important things in life!

SOME POINTS TO GET YOU GOING

1. Schedule a fitness appointment into your diary. If you treat it as an appointment, you'll have a better chance of sticking to it and this will help you avoid scheduling other things which might interfere. Be sure you make this appointment a priority. This will also help you get into the habit of exercising.

2. Exercise with a partner/or team. It's also a great way to meet new friends. When I was competing with a triathlon team I found that I worked harder. It's especially motivating when other people are counting on you. I had two other members of my team depending on me to train as hard as I could, I kept that in mind whenever I didn't feel like training, so I didn't want to let them down.

3. Start out SLOWLY, GRADUALLY and set yourself realistic goals. At first, you'll notice an improvement in your muscle tone and you'll feel more comfortable wearing exercise gear (leotards, shorts etc.), which will increase your confidence.

4. Strenuous exercise is not always necessary. Even a brisk walk has benefits, and it's a START! You'll gain a great sense of accomplishment.

EXERCISE STRENGTHENS US PHYSICALLY AND EMO-
TIONALLY and
IT'S GREAT FOR THE SPIRIT!
'THERE IS NOTHING THAT STOPS US EXCEPT OUR-
SELVES'
Peter L. Powers M.D. IDDM 29 years (accomplished marathon runner)

In a medical sense there are 4 long lasting beneficial effects of exercise.

1. Blood sugar control: working muscles take up blood sugar more readily than when they are at rest.

2. Weight control: exercising helps eliminate excess fat tissue.

3. Stress control: stress affects blood sugar control and in some cases it can cause it to rise. Exercising can help lower the blood sugar, give you a form of relaxation and a greater sense of well being.

4. Cardiovascular control: exercise can improve your cardiovascular strength by causing exertion to your entire system. Cardiovascular exercise (ie. swimming, cycling, jogging) works all of the body's major muscle groups: legs, arms, stomach, and 'the big one': the heart. With this type of exercise you are strengthening the heart and improving the efficiency of your heart thus improving the blood flow to all parts of the body. Improved blood circulation can lead to fewer problems of cold feet and hands.

Also a life-style that includes physical activity may reduce the risks of developing long-term complications.

Apart from the obvious physical benefits to keep you motivated to exercise are several others related to your personal well being. You can use the time to completely 'unwind'. You can use this as YOUR time to think, to relax, and to spend private time on your own without distracting disturbances. The saying 'Healthy body, healthy mind' comes into play here. By the same token, if you choose to socialise, this is the perfect opportunity to meet new friends or spend time with a special friend.

15

Getting Started

IT'S NEVER TOO LATE TO START AN EXERCISE
PROGRAMME

ANYONE CAN BENEFIT – AT ANY AGE

First and foremost, please consult your physician before starting an exercise programme. Especially if you've had diabetes for 10 years or more. No one should start an exercise programme without speaking with their diabetes nurse specialist or doctor first.

The first step to getting started is to educate yourself and
learn the basic rules. It just takes a bit of information with
guidelines to follow, some commonsense and a few sessions
of trial and error to make exercise a part of your diabetes
care.

THERE ARE NO SPECIFIC RULES, JUST GUIDELINES

Exercise is important, but not always easy. If you're starting
an exercise programme for the first time, chances are your
diabetes control will change. With time and practice, you'll
get it right and you'll feel that much better.

There are numerous problems (that can be overcome) for
people who exercise, unfortunately, they are all too often used
as excuses rather than hurdles, not to participate. So ... – read
on.

Before you start an exercise programme there are several
questions you need to ask yourself:

– How much time can I devote to training? e.g. 1 hour a day,
3 days per week
– What are my goals? e.g. to lose weight, run a marathon,
improve fitness level

– What time of day is the most suitable for me to exercise?
– What type of exercise do I enjoy?
– Do I want to join a team sport or do an individual sport?

First and foremost, surround yourself with people who like to exercise, they'll help keep you motivated. A 'couch potato' won't encourage you to play football or join a badminton class.

If you're not into any particular sport and would like to be, I suggest taking a shopping spree with exercise. Try several new sports and you're bound to find one you like. Check out group sessions, team sports, or rent some sports equipment and try something new: e.g. roller-blades or a mountain bike, before you invest money in something you won't stick with.

I'm not a natural athlete and never really had it in me to compete or even to participate. It wasn't until I found a sport I thoroughly enjoyed, that I was motivated enough to continue.

NOTHING VENTURED – NOTHING GAINED

As we are all creatures of habit, getting started may be difficult because you are breaking your normal routine. Start gradually and set yourself some realistic goals, both long-term and short-term. Set CLEAR goals and it'll give you a feeling of success when you achieve them. Set small goals at first and progress from there. You must approach fitness with the right ATTITUDE. Be positive and realistic. You may find it difficult to keep up with your new routine and get discouraged because of all the trial and error involved with trying to manage your diabetes and exercise.

Try not to get too discouraged, even when every muscle in your body aches and you're not seeing immediate results. Be patient, it will take time and effort and eventually you'll get it right. Don't give up too soon! Give yourself time. Listen to your own body and set your own pace. Remember that the longer you have been inactive, the longer it will take for you to restore yourself to fitness. This is another good reason to stay fit and keep exercising.

It's often a good idea to have a fitness assessment before you start a new programme. This often consists of body composition (fat measurement), tests for blood pressure, heart rate, strength, flexibility and cardiovascular stamina. Then 3 months later have a further assessment as this will enable you to see any improvements you've made and also will show you what areas you can still improve on. It will evaluate your current fitness level thus making it easier for you to adjust your programme to keep the momentum of your improvement up. When it's on paper, it's very encouraging and will help keep you motivated.

Choose a sport you'll enjoy. Whether it be for the joy of competing, finishing an exercise session or class, or beating your personal best. Make sure it's appropriate to your abilities and life-style. Exercise shouldn't be endured – but enjoyed. Above all, you must have FUN!! and if you want to get fit, GET STARTED!!

CROSS TRAINING is an excellent option. This simply means training in several different sports; i.e. running, cycling and swimming or rowing, cycling and step aerobics. This combines several activities for a balance of cardiovascular fitness, muscle strength, flexibility and endurance. The great advantage to cross training is that it helps alleviate boredom by providing diversity and stimulation. It can make exercising more interesting which helps you stick with it. You can perform different sports, which means a different challenge on alternate days. It's also excellent for training different muscle groups as each sport works different muscles.

Joining a fitness centre/health club is another good option as they usually have a number of different sports you can choose from; e.g. squash, dance classes, aerobics, weight training, swimming.

Before you purchase a membership to a club there are several things you should consider:

1. Make certain you feel comfortable in the surroundings and you like the atmosphere.
2. The location of the club is convenient to your home or work. If it's not at a suitable location you'll be less motivated

to make the journey there on the days you don't particularly feel like training.

3. Check for yourself whether the fitness instructors are fully qualified with current qualifications. Fitness techniques are constantly changing and progressing. Look at how aerobics has changed over the past decade. At the beginning of the Jane Fonda revolution it was a lot of bouncing while performing straight leg stretches. Today's current aerobic techniques are low impact cardiovascular methods and gentle stretches. Instructors should hold qualifications from reputable organisations: RSA, ACE, ACSM, AFAA or hold a degree in sports sciences or physical education.

4. And last but not least, the bottom line with fitness centres, can you afford the membership fees?

GENERAL GUIDELINES

1. CONSISTENCY: establish an exercise habit. You take your insulin and eat your meals at approximately the same times each day. Why not incorporate exercise into this type of routine?

insulin

exercise   diet

They all complement each other, one doesn't substitute another. Exercise alone is not the key to good diabetes management. It is the appropriate balancing of diet, insulin and exercise that bring the many positive benefits.

2. Exercise when blood sugar is rising, one or two hours after a meal, not when insulin is peaking. It's a good idea to eat a high-carbohydrate snack before exercising (e.g. half of a peanut butter sandwich). Avoid alcohol as it can promote low blood sugar.

3. Test your blood sugar before, during and after exercise to help prevent hypos. It is especially important to test after exercise to prevent delayed-onset hypoglycemia (post exerise hypo) which can occur as long as 6 to 15 hours after exercise.

4. Do not give your insulin injection into the exercising muscle. Exercise can increase the efficiency of the insulin uptake.

5. Note that you may have to reduce your insulin level according to the duration and intensity of the exercise. The effects of physical activity can last for up to 24 hours, therefore you may need to reduce insulin not only on the day of strenuous exercise but also on the day after.

6. Wear comfortable, appropriate footwear and clothing.

7. Make sure your exercise partner knows how to recognise the symptoms of a hypo and how to treat one.

8. All exercise sessions should include the following:

– 5–10 minute warm up before exercise – stretching. This helps the body prepare for what's about to happen!

– 30–40 minute training – cardiovascular work (this is the most vigorous activity) i.e. aerobics, cycling

– 5–10 minute cool down after exercise – stretching and relaxation. This allows the heart rate to slow down and brings the body back to its normal resting state safely. (Warm ups and cool downs can help prevent injuries.

9. Avoid exercise when ill or when diabetes control is poor.

10. ALWAYS carry appropriate treatment for hypos, i.e. Dextro Energy tablets are convenient – in case of an emergency.

11. Start an exercise programme at a comfortable level and progress gradually. Gradually increase the duration and intensity of your training. Only increase your level of exertion when the exercise is becoming too easy to perform.

12. It is advised not to exercise with a low blood sugar of <5 mmol/l, as exercising can cause it to lower quickly. If the blood sugar is >17 mmol/l, exercise can speed up the onset of ketoacidosis. If you show ketones at this stage it is best to take the appropriate actions and wait before starting an exercise session.

THE COMPONENTS OF EXERCISE

TYPE OF EXERCISE

Aerobic exercise: this includes low-intensity, long duration activities that involve the repetitive use of major muscles, e.g. swimming, rowing, cycling, jogging. Aerobic activity increases the body's production of endorphins and, as a result of this, can give you the 'runner's high', also described as 'feel good' exercise.

Anaerobic exercise: is when the high intensity activity performed requires more oxygen than the body can deliver, e.g. prolonged high intensity running.

Aerobic exercises are recommended as they improve your heart and lung fitness. It's also the best type of work out to help you lose weight.

DURATION, FREQUENCY AND INTENSITY OF EXERCISE

In order to gain maximum benefits, you should exercise at least 3 to 5 times per week, with 30 to 60 minutes duration of each session. Aerobic exercise which lasts less than 20 minutes is of little cardiovascular benefit.

It is suggested that we exercise every day as this makes insulin and diet adjustment easier to control but, if you are like me, setting a more realistic goal of exercising 4 days a week might do the trick. As long as you exercise regularly, making the right adjustments to diet and insulin will be easier and you will gain a greater knowledge of how your body reacts to exercise.

Your pulse rate should be between 50–75% of maximal heart rate. Because we are all so physically different with some people fitter than others, not everyone will be able to exercise for a full 60 minutes. Start out gradually, at your own pace, until your fitness level increases. Take rests if you begin to feel short of breath.

Another way to determine your intensity level is to do the 'talking test'. This simply means if you are not able to carry on a conversation with someone while you are exercising, you're working too hard and should slow down a bit.

TIME OF DAY TO EXERCISE

To understand the best time of day for you to exercise, it's important for you to know the timing of your insulin action i.e. when it peaks and the type of food consumed. What you've eaten may be absorbed into the blood stream quickly or slowly, causing a gradual blood sugar rise or a sudden one.

Exercising in the morning is recommended as the best time of day to exercise. It can help prevent post-exercise hypos and have the greatest impact on maintaining blood sugar levels during the day. Exercise after eating a snack and before taking your morning insulin.

Exercising in the evening can bring on a hypo while you're sleeping, due to a post-exercise hypo. This is why it is recommended to test your blood sugar before you go to bed and sometime during the evening.

The best way around all of this it seems, is to exercise at approximately the same time each day. This is especially true when you first start exercising because you're just learning about how your body reacts to it. As far as your blood sugar levels are concerned, the best time to exercise is shortly after a meal, when your blood sugar is on the rise. This will help to maintain blood sugar levels.

CONTROVERSY

Originally regular exercise was thought to improve the overall well-being in individuals with diabetes. Later it was thought to improve long-term blood sugar control. Studies today fail to prove any long-term improvement. The reason for this difference may be because of the increased caloric intake, which usually goes with exercising to prevent hypos. This may undermine any long-term positive effects of exercise on blood sugar. Exercising can cause swings between low and high blood sugars, this can give you problems if you don't try and find a happy balance.

Although this may be the case, doctors are in agreement that the benefits of regular exercise far outweigh any negatives.

RISKS

– blood sugar can drop too low during and after exercise
– already high blood sugar (>17 mmol/l) from a lack of insulin, can increase with exercise, it can also bring on ketoacidosis.
– high intensity exercise can cause blood sugar to rise
– blood pressure may rise

– risk of complications may be increased if you have unknown pre-existing complications. Another good reason to seek guidance and get tested by your nurse or doctor before starting an exercise programme.

16

Exercise and Blood Sugar Levels

!!! ADRENALIN RUSHES !!!

Adrenalin is a hormone that stimulates the nervous system.

Adrenalin rushes, in relation to exercise and diabetes, are precipitated by the fear of hypoglycemia and the nerves and excitement of competition. I'll never forget the first time I competed in a triathlon. I started the day with an average blood sugar reading, and an hour before the competition was about to begin I did another blood sugar reading and I was SKY HIGH!. Little did I know that my excitement (and nerves!) would trigger an adrenalin rush that would cause my blood sugar to rise.

Adrenalin releases glucose from the liver into the blood stream and this in turn causes the blood sugar to rise. If your blood sugar control is good, and you have taken a sufficient amount of insulin, you shouldn't be in great danger of developing hyperglycemia (as the extra sugar will be used in the exercise you're about to do). It is advised NOT to take extra insulin in anticipation of this natural blood sugar rise pre-competition, especially if you're participating in an endurance event.

ADRENALIN WILL PRODUCE AN INSULIN REACTION TYPE OF FEELING but in actual fact your blood sugar will be rising rapidly rather than dropping.

HYPERGLYCEMIA AFTER EXERCISE

There are several reasons why you could see an increase in your blood sugar after you exercise.

– adrenalin rush (as mentioned above).

– insufficient insulin and poor control. This can lead to developing ketones > ketoacidosis > coma. Make sure your diabetes is in control before you take up exercise. Consult your doctor or diabetes specialist nurse for guidance.

– you have eaten too much food in anticipation of burning it off during exercise, and to prevent a hypo. It's easy to go over board in anticipation of the energy you're going to use up and like most of us with diabetes, the last thing you want when you're exercising is a hypo creeping around the corner. It's best to work this out sensibly and bring extra glucose with you, just in case. It is not advised to eat extra food if your pre-exercise level is high or if you're exercising for a short time.

BLOOD SUGAR LEVELS

– if your blood sugar reading is >17 mmol/l or shows ketones, delay exercise until these readings improve. Exercise can cause your blood sugar to go higher and worsen the situation – you could develop ketoacidosis.

– if your blood sugar reading is <6.5 mmol/l you should take 25–50 g of carbo, at the start of moderate to heavy exercise, then take 10–15 g every ½–1 hr and monitor blood sugar.

– if your blood sugar reading is 6.5–17 mmol/l, take proportionately less carbohydrates at the start and adjust on-going intake according to test results.

FACTORS DETERMINING BLOOD SUGAR RESPONSE TO EXERCISE:

DECREASE IN BLOOD SUGAR IF:

– too much insulin exists during exercise
– exercise lasts more than 60 min. or intensive exercise longer than 30 min.
– more than 3 hrs. since your last meal
– no extra snacks are taken before or during exercise.

INCREASE IN BLOOD SUGAR IF:

– lack of insulin exists during exercise
– exercise is strenuous
– excessive carbohydrates taken before or during exercise

BLOOD SUGAR REMAINS UNCHANGED IF:

– exercise is short
– plasma insulin concentration is adequate
– appropriate snacks are taken before and during exercise

** 2 hours of vigorous exercise can change your blood sugar control for more than 24 hours whereas moderate exercise can change control for 1–2 hours.

KETONES

To test for ketones, you simply take a 'Ketostix' strip (reagent strips for urinalysis – available from your G.P. on prescription), dip it into a fresh specimen of urine, then compare the test strip colour to the corresponding colour chart on the bottle to determine what your ketone level is.

The presence of ketones may indicate a state of starvation. In individuals with diabetes a lack of insulin can produce ketones. What happens is the body's cells send messages that they are starving, causing more energy to be sent from the liver. The absence of insulin means that the blood sugar cannot be taken up by the body's cells. The blood sugar then rises, but the cells are still saying they're starving so ketones develop at a faster rate. Large amounts of ketones are dangerous, and if this goes unchecked, it can lead to ketoacidosis (an acid condition of the blood) and ultimately death.

What to look out for:
1. Ketones with high blood sugar: this often happens to individuals with poorly controlled diabetes. Vigorous exercise can actually produce ketones. However, it is dangerous if we exercise when we have ketones and high blood sugar due to a lack of insulin. The first thing you need to do is look at your overall control. Then to treat this you should take insulin, consume extra carbohydrates, measure your blood sugar at frequent intervals and keep testing urine for ketones until

your result is negative and your blood sugar is at a controlled level.

2. High blood sugar without ketones: on a short-term basis this is not too dangerous, but it should not continue for long periods of time. This can be treated with exercise or a small dose of short-acting insulin.

17

Reactions/Hypos & Hypers

'HITTING THE WALL'
(Long distance athletes term for running out of fuel)

None of us are immune to our 'little side-kicks', universally known as 'hypos'. You mustn't take the attitude that a hypo won't/can't happen to YOU. You probably know by now, denial of having a hypo when you are actually having one, is one of the symptoms of low blood sugar. Hypos affect us physically and emotionally. Everyone reacts differently. I, for one, get quiet, withdrawn, moody and short-tempered. This of course should not be used as an excuse to be difficult to get along with. Just as the threat of hypos/hypers shouldn't be used as an excuse not to participate in exercise or competition.

Low blood sugar reactions (< 4mmol/l) affect athletic performance in a number of ways.

– reduction in co-ordination ability (ie. not able to hit the tennis ball from the correct angle)
– increase in response time
– inability to concentrate
– general feeling of fatigue – this can lower enthusiasm.

You can reduce the fear of hypos by seeing if you can identify a distinctive pattern of symptoms. Remember that not everyone's symptoms are exactly the same.

How to avoid a hypo during exercise:

– reduce insulin and /or increase diet – consume extra food (usually carbos). This may be required before, during, or after exercise.
Things to consider:

– time of last meal or snack taken and what it consisted of
– intensity and duration of exercise
– insulin action (when is your insulin peaking?)
– injection site
– monitoring blood sugars
– avoid exercise immediately before a meal
– take extra carbos before and during prolonged exercise
– weather – ambient temperature.

Note that making changes is a very individual thing and what works for one athlete may not necessarily work for another. What I have listed are guidelines to follow.

TREATING HYPOS DURING EXERCISE

Stop exercising if you feel a hypo coming on and treat it immediately. If you're participating in a team sport, make sure someone knows how to correctly assist you.

Some quick acting and convenient forms of treatment are as follows:

– Dextro Energy tablets
– fruit juice is the quickest way to increase blood sugar level, especially if it's fibre free. Fibre will slow down the uptake and action of fructose in the juice. Ice cream, sweets, chocolate are not a good choice because of their high fat content. Fat slows down the absorption of sugar which means it would take longer for your blood sugar to rise.

If consciousness is lost, someone can help you by placing glucose gel under your tongue, or glucagon can be injected into your arm, this will stimulate your liver to produce glucose.

The time it takes for you to resume exercise depends on a number of things: intensity of exercise, how low the blood sugar was, the speed of action of the food/drink taken.

BLOOD SUGAR MONITORING

1. Monitor blood sugar immediately before, during (every 30 minutes) and 15 minutes after exercise. Monitor blood sugar at night and take additional carbohydrates prior to sleep.
2. Delay exercise if blood sugar is 11.5 mmol/l or higher and ketones are present.
3. Consume carbohydrates if blood sugar is less than 5 mmol/l.
4. Learn individual blood sugar response to different types of exercise.
5. Avoid exercising late at night. Exercise earlier in the day, reduce evening insulin dose after exercise is performed.

Frequent blood sugar monitoring will help keep you in better control as the results will show you the effects of exercise on your blood sugar.

by Barbara Campaigne PhD

EVERYONE SHOULD BE FAMILIAR WITH THE WAYS TO DETECT AND TREAT HYPOGLYCEMIA AND HYPERGLYCEMIA

TREATING HYPOS BEFORE EXERCISE

To ward off a reaction during exercise, it's important to make sure your blood sugar level is high enough before exercising. There is no magic level for everyone to follow, there are so many factors involved and with time, trial and error, you will find what level works best for you. If you are low, take some quick acting carbohydrates (approx. 10 gms), wait for 15 –30 minutes before you exercise. You must allow time for the sugar to be digested and absorbed into the blood. Then before you start, test your blood sugar again to make sure there is an increase.

Start exercising on a gentle level, then gradually build up and if you're in any doubt as to whether your blood sugar is going down a bit, do another blood test and act accordingly. This isn't the day to push yourself to the maximum. Don't forget to test your blood sugar after you exercise. If your sugar is low, take extra carbohydrates. If it is high, do not take extra insulin as you'll just be creating a see-saw effect. Remember, you'll still be burning energy after you stop exercising.

EARLY WARNING SIGNS OF LOW BLOOD SUGARS (HYPOGLYCEMIA)

RAPID ONSET:

– headache, hunger, fatigue, nervousness, numbness, slurred speech, irritability, perspiration, sometimes feelings of not caring and being emotionally upset.

** during exercise you need to learn the difference between exercise fatigue and an actual hypo. It's easy to confuse the two as some of the symptoms are similar: sweating, fatigue, increased heart rate. The best way to be certain of course is to test your blood sugar.

KNOW THE WARNING SIGNS OF HIGH BLOOD SUGARS (HYPERGLYCEMIA)

SLOW ONSET:

– increased thirst, increased urination, abdominal pains, nausea, ketones in urine, lack of appetite, fruity or sweet odour on breath, feeling sleepy and lethargic.

THE SOMOGYI EFFECT

A low blood sugar can sometimes lead to a high blood sugar for hours afterwards. The somogyi effect is caused by a low blood sugar reaction followed by a high blood sugar reaction. When a low blood sugar reaction triggers the release of glucose from the liver glycogen, causing your blood sugar to rise and, combined with the sugar you've taken to treat your hypo, the end result can be a high blood sugar.

SPECIAL CONSIDERATIONS

'Sitting on the bench'

It happens to the best of us! Be prepared for if (and hopefully – when) you get called on to play. Have some quick acting carbohydrate nearby (ie. Gatorade).

18

Diet and Exercise

WEIGHTY MATTERS

My personal rule of thumb has always been: 'NEVER JUMP ON A SCALE'. The best way to measure whether or not you are losing any weight is to simply stand naked in front of your full length mirror (doing this in a dimly lit room doesn't count). The second best way to tell is by the way your clothes fit, or don't fit and you have to adjust the notches on your belt. Your goal should be to lose inches rather than weight. The reason I say this is because if you have recently started an exercise programme, chances are that you are toning and developing your muscles, losing some clay (fat), and since muscle weighs more than fat, you'll probably notice an increase rather than a decrease in your weight when you jump on the scale. This can be very discouraging if you are trying to lose or maintain your body weight.

These 'Get Thin Quick!' diets are unhealthy for anyone, especially for people who have diabetes. Incorporating exercise into your regime can help you achieve a healthier weight loss while ensuring you are developing rather than burning muscle tissue.

The two main reasons why some people gain weight after starting an exercise programme are:
a) they eat extra food in case of a hypo rather than cutting back on their insulin.
b) they over compensate with food during a hypo after an exercise session.

This is all very frustrating and counter-productive. Your first step to correct or prevent this is to work out a PERSONAL exercise programme which includes: diet, exercise, and insulin. They all work TOGETHER – exercising without cutting back on food or insulin to prevent hypos won't make it easy to lose weight. There is no set pattern for everyone to follow, like the other areas of diabetes. What works for you might not work for someone else. You'll learn how your body reacts to different levels of physical exertion. It's important to find a right balance for your blood sugars in relation to diet and exercise. As a doctor once told me 'You need to be a physician of your own body'.

If your goal is to lose weight, you'll need to work out a balance between reducing your insulin dose and cutting back on the food you eat and drink. The easiest way to make this adjustment is to be consistent and exercise at approximately the same time every day and work with your health care team on establishing a new insulin regime and diet. Note that regular exercise can reduce the amount of insulin you need by bringing your blood sugar levels down. Taking less insulin, you can reduce the amount of extra food you would need to eat or drink. Another important adjustment to make is to consider WHAT you eat and drink to treat or prevent a hypo during exercise. Fresh fruit, juice, dextrose tablets, energy drinks will all give you sugar for extra energy but without the empty calories you'd get if you consumed chocolate bars or sweet biscuits as these contain mainly fat.

Fast weight loss programmes, such as meal substitution drinks, are actually unhealthy and can cause you to lose muscle tissue, not necessarily stored fat.

EXERCISE AND DIETARY REQUIREMENTS

If one of your goals from exercising is to lose weight, you'll be pleased to discover that it plays a crucial role in successful, permanent weight loss. Contrary to popular belief, exercising actually decreases your appetite, rather than increases it.

You are not only burning calories while you are exercising, but also for many hours afterwards. Extra calories are continuing to burn once you stop exercising. This also explains why you may experience low blood sugar hours later (post-exercise hypos), and sometimes even on the day following strenuous exercise.

The adjustment of your diet with regard to carbohydrate supplements depends on: the duration and intensity of exercise; the blood sugar level before exercise; the time of day of exercise – in relation to action of insulin and prevailing insulin levels.

Do not consume large amounts of carbohydrates before exercising. It's best to eat a balanced, mixed meal including protein in order to maintain a continuous flow of energy.

If you are interested in endurance events, anything lasting over two hours, you'll need to take a closer look at your diet and carbohydrate intake. Complex carbohydrates (starch) should be your main fuel source. 'Carbo-loading', eating a low carbohydrate diet days before an event, then consuming a mass quantity the night before the event, used to be all the rage for endurance athletes. It was believed that this method increased muscle glycogen stores and enabled you to perform longer. Athletes today are claiming that maintaining a consistently high carbohydrate intake during training is more effective and equally, it's more practical for the athlete who has diabetes.

HYDRATION MANAGEMENT

– consume a litre of liquid 2 hours before an event
– 200 mls for each 20–30 minutes of activity
– 400 mls of cool water for each pound of weight loss which occurred due to exercise.

It's important to make sure you drink enough fluids before, during and after exercise to avoid dehydration. By maintaining the right amount of fluid in the body you can help regulate the amount of sugar in the blood during exercise.

Listed below are general guidelines for making food adjustments for exercise. Keep in mind that no two individuals are alike, and that there are many different factors to consider when deciding on how to make food adjustments for exercise.

GENERAL GUIDELINES FOR MAKING FOOD ADJUSTMENTS FOR EXERCISE
by Barbara Campaigne, PhD

Type of exercise and examples:	If blood glucose is:	Increase food intake by:	Suggestions of food to use:
Exercise of short duration and of low to moderate intensity.	less than 4.5 mmol/l	10 to 15 gms of carbos.	1 fruit or crunchy muesli bar e.g.Tracker, Harvest Crunch.
e.g. walking a half mile or leisurely cycling for less than 30 minutes.	4.5 mmol/l or above	not necessary to increase food	
Exercise of moderate intensity.	>4.5 mmol/l	25 to 50 gms of carbos. before exercise then 10–15 gms per hr of ex.	Milk or fruit juice plus Kit Kat or Twix or similar.
e.g. Tennis, swimming, jogging, leisurely cycling or golfing for an hour.	4.5–9.5 mmol/l	10–15 gms of carbos. per hr of exercise	1 fruit or slice of toast
	10–16.5 mmol/l	not necessary to increase food	
	>18 mmol/l	Exercise is not advised until blood sugar is under control. Check for ketones.	
Strenuous activity or exercise	<4.5 mmol/l	50 gms of carbos. monitor bg carefully	Roll plus milk or fruit juice plus a chocolate biscuit and milk.
e.g. Football, hockey, racquetball strenuous cycling, swimming. (depending on intensity & duration)	4.5–9.5 mmol/l	25–50 gms of carbos.	Fruit juice or milk plus a slice of toast.
	10–16.5 mmol/l	10–15 gms of carbos. per hour of exercise.	1 fruit or 1 bread exch.

YOU SHOULD TAKE A SUPPLEMENTAL CARBOHY-DRATE SNACK (60–90 KCAL) EVERY 30 MINUTES IF EXERCISE IS VIGOROUS.

– For cycling it may be an idea to fill your water bottle with Lucozade and to take regular small sips throughout the ride.
– It is strongly recommended that you reduce your insulin so that you don't need to eat more than about 20 grams of carbohydrate for regular exercise.
– It's important to keep your body's carbohydrate stores replenished. Carbohydrate stores in the body are limited so you should increase your complex carbohydrate intake less than 24 hours before and after exercise, depending on intensity and duration of exercise. Failing to do so may result in you not being able to exercise intensely and may also leave you feeling fatigued. It takes a minimum of 20 hours to totally replenish your body's carbohydrate stores.
– The breakfast before participating in an endurance exercise should contain 20–30g protein and approx. 40g of carbohydrates.
– During strenuous long-term exercise a carbohydrate intake of 40g/hr combined with a reduced insulin dosage.

ALCOHOL + SPORT

Since social drinking (the pub scene) is a high priority in this country, chances are you're not going to abstain just because you have diabetes. Nor should you feel that you have to. If you maintain the 'everything in moderation' attitude and a little knowledge on how to make adjustments you should be able to cope like everyone else.

It's common to have a few drinks after a rugby match and then have a low blood sugar because of the combination of exercise and alcohol.

First and foremost you must understand that:

ALCOHOL BLOCKS GLUCOSE PRODUCTION BY THE LIVER

If you are exercising all day, for example skiing, stopping at the mountain top restaurant for lunch and a couple of pints of lager and then skiing for the rest of the afternoon, a hypo may occur because the alcohol from the beer is blocking the production of glucose that's stored in your liver. The exercise has used up all of the available glucose .

CARBOHYDRATES

What are carbohydrates? It's important for individuals with diabetes to know how carbohydrates affect their blood sugar and energy levels.

Carbohydrate is a collective term for various types of sugar and starch. The various carbohydrates differ in their specific effects on blood sugar and physical performance.

Carbohydrates produce the energy needed to promote muscle activity and growth and are the primary source of fuel for muscle contraction. They are the most important nutrient for athletic performance. The energy from carbohydrates can be released to the exercising muscle up to three times quicker than the energy released from fat. Once consumed, carbohydrates travel to the liver where they may be reserved as glycogen or travel through the blood stream. Glycogen is an important source of energy. Once in the liver glycogen may be turned into glucose which is then released through the blood stream to help meet the body's increased need for energy.

It is beneficial to consume carbohydrates during competition to maximise athletic performance.

The three major groups of carbohydrates can be described as:

1. Rapidly absorbed carbohydrates = sugars
Contained in dextrose, soft drinks, various fruits and sweets.
2. Slowly absorbable carbohydrates = starch
Contained in whole wheat bread, cereals, muesli, potatoes and rice.
3. Indigestible carbohydrates = fibre (roughage)
Contained in raw fruit and vegetables, and oat bran.

In simplistic terms it can be said that carbohydrates from:

Dextrose, sucrose,
soft drinks, apple juice,　　　—>　　　shoot into the blood
energy drinks for athletes

Flour products, cereals, bread, potatoes, pastas, rice	—>	flow into the blood
Raw fruit	—>	trickle into the blood
Dairy products	—>	drip into the blood
Whole grain muesli, whole wheat/rye bread, (raw vegetable) salads, legumes, oat bran	—>	seep into the blood

by Rosemarie Brewer
(dietician)

Examples of high-carbohydrate foods are: apple sauce, banana, fruit yoghurt, spaghetti with tomato sauce, baked potato, rice, raisins.

1 gram of carbohydrate= 4kcals of energy

DIET GUIDELINES ANNOUNCED BY THE BDA

FAT 30 –35%
PROTEIN 10 –15%
CARBOHYDRATES 50%

FAT should comprise 30–35% of energy – saturated and polyunsaturated fat less than 10% of daily intake and monounsaturated fats more than 10%.

PROTEIN should make up 10–15% of total energy. People with nephropathy should reduce their protein intake.

CARBOHYDRATE 50% of total energy. Foods rich in complex carbohydrate and water soluble fibre are preferable.

Carbos are digested more rapidly when consumed alone, without protein or fat and sugar is digested more rapidly than starch.

Processed and refined foods are digested more rapidly than whole and refined foods.

Fibre in foods appear to slow down the release of energy from food. e.g. the sugar is not absorbed as quickly.

There are two main sources of fuel: carbohydrates and fat. Carbohydrates is the primary and preferred source of fuel while fat is the reserve fuel for energy.

19

Insulin

Insulin is the hormone that regulates the way sugars are used for fuel by the body. Insulin and exercise work together to use up glucose.

It's important to find a happy medium for insulin levels during exercise. If your blood insulin level is too low, exercise can make the situation worse. As your muscles start to exercise they begin to draw glucose from the blood and as the blood sugar level falls, your brain sends a signal to your liver, which sends an emergency supply of glucose to your blood, thus causing your blood sugarlevel to raise too high – no matter how much exercise you do.

To avoid this, check blood sugar before exercise. If it is >17 mmol/l, check urine for ketones and if present, postpone exercise. Take short-acting insulin as required. The amount of insulin depends on many variables. Frequent blood sugar monitoring will give insight into this. The correct blood insulin level can keep the blood sugar steady during exercise as long as liver stores of glycogen are adequate.

If you are not consuming excessive carbos and your blood sugar increases during exercise then you should increase your insulin dose slightly or change your insulin schedule in order to have enough insulin on board during exercise.

INSULIN ADJUSTMENTS

The insulin dose to be reduced is the insulin that will be peaking during the time of exercise.

Multiple injections: reduce short-acting insulin taken before exercise by 30–50 %. You should never change the long-acting insulin dose. If exercise lasts for several hours take extra carbos during exercise

Keeping a record of your past experiences in an exercise diary will assist you in making correct decisions regarding insulin and diet to co-ordinate with your exercise routine. Through trial and error, experience and regular review of your diary, you will learn how, where and when to make adjustments.

1. Decrease the insulin dose:
a) intermediate-acting insulin: decrease by 30–35% on the day of exercise
b) intermediate and short-acting insulin: omit dose of short-acting insulin that precedes exercise
c) multiple doses of short-acting insulin: reduce the dose prior to exercise by 30–50% and supplement carbohydrates
d) continuous subcutaneous infusion: eliminate meal time bolus or increment that precedes or immediately follows exercise
2. DO NOT EXERCISE AT THE TIME OF PEAK INSULIN ACTION.

When exercise coincides with the peak insulin action, the glucose production from the liver cannot increase sufficiently to match the exercise induced increase in muscle glucose uptake therefore leading to a severe hypo during or after exercise.

Ideally, exercise when insulin will not be peaking and with a blood glucose level of 6.5–11 mmol/l. In this situation glucose uptake by the muscle is matched by liver glucose production therefore a hypo is avoided.

Overestimating and underestimating the amount of insulin required is always a possibility. Following these guidelines should make this challenge a little easier.

ABSORPTION RATE OF INSULIN

The arms and stomach have the quickest absorption rate followed by:

legs
buttocks

Never give your insulin injection into the exercising muscle. In other words, if you are going cycling, you give your insulin injection in the arm and not the legs as they are the main muscles being used in this sport. If you give the insulin injection into active muscles, blood flow will cause a rapid absorption of the insulin. Always inject insulin into the areas of low muscle activity.

INSULIN PEAK ACTION TIMES

Preparation		Manufacturer	Species	Onset, peak activity and duration of action in hours (approx) 0 2 4 6 8 10 12 14 16 18 20 22 24 26 28 30 32 34
Neutral Insulin Injection	Actrapid (pyr)	Novo Nordisk		
	Human Velosulin (emp)	Novo Nordisk		
	Humulin S (prb)	Lilly		
	Hypurin Neutral	CP Pharm		
	Velosulin	Novo Nordisk		
Biphasic Insulin Injection*	Human Actraphane (pyr)	Novo Nordisk		
	Human Initard 50/50 (emp)	Novo Nordisk		
	Human Mixtard 30/70 (emp)	Novo Nordisk		
	Humulin M1 (prb)	Lilly		
	Humulin M2 (prb)	Lilly		
	Humulin M3 (prb)	Lilly		
	Humulin M4 (prb)	Lilly		
	Humulin M5 (prb)	Lilly		
	Initard 50/50	Novo Nordisk		
	Mixtard 30/70	Novo Nordisk		
	PenMix 10/90 (pyr)	Novo Nordisk		
	PenMix 20/80 (pyr)	Novo Nordisk		
	PenMix 30/70 (pyr)	Novo Nordisk		
	PenMix 40/60 (pyr)	Novo Nordisk		
	PenMix 50/50 (pyr)	Novo Nordisk		
	Rapitard MC	Novo Nordisk	25% + 75%	
Insulin Zinc Suspension (Amorphous)	Semitard MC	Novo Nordisk		
Isophane Insulin Injection	Human Insulatard (emp)	Novo Nordisk		
	Human Protaphane (pyr)	Novo Nordisk		
	Humulin I (prb)	Lilly		
	Hypurin Isophane	CP Pharm		
	Insulatard	Novo Nordisk		
Insulin Zinc Suspension (Mixed)	Human Monotard (pyr)	Novo Nordisk		
	Humulin Lente (prb)	Lilly		
	Hypurin Lente	CP Pharm		
	Lentard MC	Novo Nordisk	30% + 70%	
Insulin Zinc Suspension (Crystalline)	Human Ultratard (pyr)	Novo Nordisk		
	Humulin Zn (prb)	Lilly		
Protamine Zinc Insulin Injection	Hypurin Protamine Zinc	CP Pharm		

(prb)-produced from proinsulin synthesised by bacteria using recombinant DNA technology
(pyr)-produced from a precursor synthesised by yeast using recombinant DNA technology
(emp)-produced by enzymatic modification of porcine insulin
*Speed of onset is proportional to amount of soluble insulin

It's very important to know the action time of the insulins you are taking in order to make the appropriate adjustments.
Reproduced by: MIMS, Haymarket Medical Ltd.
Please note that this chart is updated monthly.

20

The 'Diabetics Bible': Daily Diary

Included in your diary should be:

– BLOOD SUGAR and ketone urinalysis results
– EXERCISE: duration (i.e. ½ day skiing), type of exercise (i.e. 2 km cycle), intensity (i.e. competition day)
– TIME of day (use the exact time – not simply am/pm – exercise was performed, blood sugar taken, and when food was eaten
– INSULIN: dose and type
– Injection site used
– DIET: type of meal/snack
– HYPOS: record any hypos and what was used to treat them. If your reactions frequently result in the Somogyi Effect (a low blood sugar followed by a high blood sugar), your nurse/ doctor will need to see this recorded so they can help you adjust your insulin dose appropriately. If this is not recorded, they may prescribe an increase in your insulin dose when it really needs a decrease.
– GENERAL HEALTH: note if you have a cold, the flu, menstrual cycle or anything that could affect your performance or blood sugar results.

(You should develop your own code system of abbreviations to record information in your diary).

With this important information recorded you and your health care team can see what is happening and then make the appropriate adjustments necessary. It will enable you to make educated guesses rather than trying to rely on your memory for all the details. You'll also be able to learn from your experiences so you don't consistently have the same problems. You'll be able to see similarities and differences in your results and this will help you to prepare for the next time. It's important to realise that there are answers for most, if not all, of the problems. The more detailed your information the better you'll be able to make the correct choices. Make sure you keep honest and accurate records and, remember, you're doing this for YOURSELF!

By including the exercise you've done, it can also act as a motivator by giving you a real sense of accomplishment.

21

Diabetic Complications and Exercise

Exercise is for everyone to enjoy and benefit from. If you suffer from a diabetes related complication, it's no excuse to be inactive. There are just a few modifications you'll need to make. The first thing you must do is have a thorough medical examination from your diabetes specialist. You must also be stabilised with your medication, diet and any other treatment that's required, e.g. dialysis, laser treatment.

ACTIVE PROLIFERATIVE RETINOPATHY:

As you are more prone to bleeding, you should avoid strenuous, high intensity exercise that causes an increase in blood pressure. A rise in blood pressure can cause pressure against the weakened blood vessels in your eyes, which could increase the risk of damage to your retina by causing a haemorrhage. Exercises to avoid would be weight lifting, jogging, rowing, and any type of exercise which promotes jarring, bouncing motions. Using 'gravity boots' and performing stretching or abdominal exercises while hanging upside down or bent over at the waist, are also not advisable.

If your proliferative retinopathy is not in an active stage and you still insist on weight lifting, make sure you go about it in an intelligent fashion. Proper breathing and close monitoring of your blood pressure is essential. The breathing technique to use is: exhale when you lift the weight, and inhale when you lower the weight. Low weights and frequent repetitions are recommended, you should be able to complete a minimum of 15 repetitions per set without too much fatigue. If not, lower the amount of weights you're lifting. Recommended sports are: cycling; road and stationary bicycles, swimming, walking, jogging, low-impact aerobics, and swimming.

If you've recently undergone laser treatment or vitrectomy surgery, it's advised to perform only mild exercise during the first 3 weeks (walking is excellent). Avoid any sport which causes jolting or jarring movements, such as: running, racquet sports, and weight lifting. Swimming should also be avoided during this period as there is an increased danger of infection and irritation into your eyes from the recent operation. With this condition intense weight training should be avoided at all costs, as it applies a great strain on the head causing too much pressure which could lead to serious damage as far as diabetic retinopathy goes. It simply is not worth the risk.

After the three week rest period following treatment, providing there are no further complications, you may commence an exercise programme slowly and GRADUALLY. Pace yourself and increase your level of exertion over a period of time (6–8 weeks). Golfing is highly recommended and you can increase the level of exertion by not using a golf cart (or a caddy!)

If your vision is impaired, the exercise options open to you have greatly expanded and progressed in the last few years. If your vision is severely impaired, some of the more popular exercise options to try are:

Swimming: is an excellent all round sport as it builds strength and improves your cardiovascular system. It requires minimal assistance from an exercise partner, as you can use buoys and ropes to divide the lanes in the swimming pool and your partner can tap you on the head with a sponge ball to let you know you've reached the end of the lane.

Jogging: on an outdoor track; a guide can assist by touching forearms slightly as you move side by side, or use a short rope between the two of you to maintain contact. In an indoor track, a wire can be used as guidance and allow for more independence.

Snow-skiing: this sport has become very popular for the visually impaired with blind athletes who have diabetes participating in the Disabled Olympics. Skiing may be accomplished through the use of a sighted partner and he/she can verbally guide you down the ski slope.

RENAL NEPHROPATHY:

Individuals on hemodialysis will benefit from aerobic activities such as: brisk walking, swimming and cycling. Intensity for this type of work out should be 60–80% of your maximum heart rate. Like all exercise, you should attempt this at a gradual level working up to a goal of prolonged endurance. Note that fluid replacement may be required if exercising in heat or following dialysis treatment. Be cautious of post-exercise hypos from the combined effects of the hemodialysis and exercise and of keeping your blood pressure at a controlled level. It is known that constant high blood pressure accelerates diabetic nephropathy.

SENSORIMOTOR NEUROPATHY:

Symptoms of this condition include: impaired balance, numbness, loss of touch, body awareness and joint position sense. Daily movement to the major joints; hip, ankles, knees, shoulders, elbows is essential to prevent shortening of the muscles. These movements should be performed gently so as not to over-stretch the muscles. You should stop the exercise if you experience any pain. If you experience any loss of sensation to your feet, the best way to prevent problems from occurring is by wearing appropriate footwear and changing your shoes on a regular basis. This would help in the distribution of your body weight by placing less stress on the same areas of your feet. It's also important to inspect your feet after exercising for any blisters, or redness. This should be a part of every diabetics daily routine.

AUTONOMIC NEUROPATHY:

For individuals with this type of neuropathy, you may become easily fatigued with little exertion. You should cease exercising if you are unable to carry on a conversation or are having trouble maintaining pedalling motions on the bicycle. It is especially important for you to consume adequate fluids before, during, and after exercise. Water exercises and stationary cycling are good exercise options to try. Swimming is particularly beneficial as the pressure of the water surrounding the body helps maintain blood pressure. Exercise activities to avoid are intense running, callisthenic exercises that require sudden changes in body position.

PERIPHERAL VASCULAR DISEASE:

Research has showed that individuals with peripheral vascular disease greatly benefit from long term exercise. Exercise options to try are: swimming, walking on a treadmill (slowly), stationary cycling. If you are in a wheelchair, or have lost a limb, chair exercises (upper body exercises) are an excellent option as well as wheelchair racing, swimming, skiing, basketball, and archery. If you experience any pain during exercise, decrease the intensity of your training and allow for periods of rest.

If the circulation in your feet and legs is poor you may experience leg pain or cramping, usually at night. Walking is a beneficial treatment, start out slowly and make sure you attempt to continue walking at the first few signs of discomfort. If you keep walking you'll encourage circulation by allowing the smaller blood vessels to open up and encourage an alternative route. If the pain is too great, slow down or stop and resume once the pain subsides.

Training Partners –
The International Diabetic Athletes Association

Unquestionably the best person to train with is a friend who also has diabetes. They will be able to recognise a potential problem and know how to cope with it in the most efficient way. They'll help you treat it and then get on with things.

I also find that training with another diabetic gives you an added sense of security knowing that they know exactly what to do. They can also relate to what you are experiencing and therefore appreciate the extra things that go with having diabetes and performing in sports.

The International Diabetic Athletes Association is an excellent organisation to get people with diabetes in contact with others that are interested in sports.

Whoever you choose for an exercise partner, make sure they know your warning signs of a hypo and how to take the appropriate steps.

CLEARING THE HURDLES TO SAFE EXERCISE

by Paula Harper RN, CDE
(Founder of the International Diabetic Athletes
Association)

I embarked on a running progam in 1976 with little information about how it would affect my type I diabetes. I developed a training regimen to build my endurance and withing a year entered my first marathon race. I went on to complete 30 more marathons, one ultramarathon (50 miles), as well as five triathlons and six century (100 plus miles) bicycle races.

Now that was quite an athletic feat for someone who previously wasn't big on exercise. The problem came when I sought medical advice for training. I was most often told not to do it or given inadequate or misleading advice. My heritage is German, so being told no was not about to stop me...... stubborn is what my husband calls me. I was troubled to learn that doctors had little helpful advice and were gernerally unwilling to work with me.

I set out on training runs, kept good records to chart my progress, and learned the most by 'trial and error'. In retrospect, what I did seems scary. These were the days before home blood sugar monitoring, and I am sure there were times when I exercised with my blood sugar too high or low. With miles to go in one marathon, I had exhausted my supply of sugar-containing snacks and was experiencing low blood sugar due to poor advice by my physician regarding the amount of insulin to take for this endurance event, I was urged to drop out of the race. I wouldn't think of it. Someone at an aid station gave me a soda, a policeman handed me a pack of chewing gum and I crossed the finish line feeling better than I had in the middle. Granted, this is not the optimal plan for running a 26 mile distance, but it worked. I wasn't fast, but I was never a quitter.

I RUN ON INSULIN became my byword . . . I had it printed on the back of a t-shirt and to my surprise, when I wore it in races, I made many new friends who also had diabetes and endured similar problems. This growing network of active people with diabetes was actually the first step in starting this organization. I came to learn of many young athletes who were being kept from participation due to coaches fears of difficulties with blood sugar regulation and I realized the big need for education and the crime in turning off youngsters to sports. I feel that the characteristics that allow an athlete to compete successfully and those needed to maintain good blood glucose control are essentially identical.

a. The **desire** to do the job right (the ability to make a short and long range commitment to continually learn about the disease and make the necessary adjustment in life style that are required for excellent glucose control).

b. An **understanding** of how the game is played and what

must be done to succeed (detailed knowledge about the pathophysiology of diabetes, the various types of insulin and their actions, the effect of diet and exercise on blood sugar regulation).

c. The **discipline** to consistently do what is needed to succeed (to methodically monitor blood glucose multiple times daily, to avoid unhealthy diet and activity patterns while making healthy alternatives a routine part of one's daily life).

d. **Skill** (the ability to accurately check blood glucose and to choose the appropriate dietary manipulations to prevent major swings in blood glucose before, during, and after exercise).

The person with diabetes who lacks these qualities is doomed to failure on and off the athletic field. On the other hand, it is possible that in some, the attraction of athletic success together with the appropriate support of coaches, physicians, and family, may provide the necessary means for developing the qualities in an otherwise stubborn youngster. By the same token, these qualities may be more evident but inadequately developed in other young diabetics who wish to participate in sports. Again, the appropriate support system can do much to help with the development of both diabetes management and athletic skills in these individuals. I knew that it was possible to provide encouragement, support and education to the growing number of individuals with diabetes.

I guess it was that determination that spurred me to go the distance in fulfilling a dream I had of encouraging other individuals with diabetes to make regular exercise a part of their daily lives and provide education about the risks and benefits. Interviewing a number of people with and without diabetes, I found that more than anything, regular physical activity makes a person feel good. It is true that exercising with diabetes demands some juggling but it is all worth the effort required to my way of thinking.

I contacted Clifton Bogardus, MD, Chief of the NIDDK Clinical Diabetes and Nutrition Section of the National Institutes of Health and Ed Horton, MD, professor and Chairman of the Department of Medicine at the University of Vermont College of Medicine, and immediate past president of the American Diabetes Association. These men have done extensive research with individuals with Type I and II diabetes and exercise. They agreed that there was a need and assisted me in making national and international contacts. In the formative stage, I met some senior executives from Squibb-Novo who, likewise, indicated that this information was essential and needed on an international level.

We went to the American Diabetes Association and worked to form a Professional Council on Exercise, to help spread our enthusiasm and address the concerns and risks involved. This all started in 1985. Doctors Horton and Bogardus and I held the first offices that made up this Council. A Position Statement on safe exercise was published this year which gives basic guidelines. The Council worked long and hard to come up with the appropriate information.

We have grown by word of mouth for the most part. I am pleased by the support we have got from professional diabetic athletes like Jonathan Hayes, tight end for the Kansas City Chiefs, Curt Fraser, former left wing for the Chicago Blackhawks and Minnesota NorthStars – now coaching the Milwaukee Admirals Hockey Team, Clive Caldwell, Canadian professional Squash player, and Scott Verplank, winner of the 1988 US Open Golf tournament. I see real evidence of a team spirit – local chapters in the United States and Canada, and affiliated groups abroad are growing and expanding. Jean-Jacques Grimm, MD and Professor Michael Berger, MD have been instrumental in the development of IDAA in Europe. Our purpose statement reads as follows:

The International Diabetic Athletes Association (IDAA) is an independent, non-profit organization of persons with diabetes and interested health professionals which is dedicated to:
– providing opportunities for the open sharing of information and skills necessary for successfully integrating diabetes and a vigorous lifestyle
– promoting participation by individuals with diabetes in sports activities
– promoting networking and support among athletes with diabetes
– providing educational opportunities for athletes with diabetes to enhance self care skills and quality of life

– providing educational opportunities to increase awareness and skill of health care professionals who counsel active people with diabetes.

Beginning in 1988, we have held annual conferences to bring together health care professionals and individuals with diabetes to hear the latest in pertinent information from an honored faculty of researchers and clinicians and also to learn from each other. All too often, it's the lack of specific information on balancing exercise and diabetes that keeps primary care physicians from encouraging patients with diabetes to participate in vigorous sports. On all levels, there is a tremendous need for education. We conduct workshops in a wide variety of sports, each led by diabetic athletes, to help people learn and address specific questions about blood sugar control with various activities.

A quarterly newsletter is published for members in four languages. Recent topics include post exercise, late onset, hypoglycemia and the values and risks of carbohydrate loading as well as information on exercise like gardening and wood cutting and how they can burn calories and need to be reckoned with. To date, there are publications in the US, Germany, French speaking Europe (Switzerland, France, Belgium, Luxembourg) and Barcelona, Spain. New groups have recently formed in Italy and Japan. We are truly developing a global network of diabetic athletes.

APPENDICES

Contributed Articles

*Thank you to Paula Harper and the IDAA
for the following articles*

Britain's Ambassador

*'Whatever you want to do, be it in sports, academics, or your profes-
sional life, go out and do it – don't let diabetes stand in your way. Let
diabetes live with you rather than let it rule your life.'*

Gary Mabbutt MBE

Ever since Gary was a child he dreamed of playing football and of
playing for his country. After all, it was in his blood. Both his father
and big brother were outstanding players. His football career started
in 1978 with the Third Division Bristol Rovers.

It was December 1978 when Gary developed an unquenchable
thirst, multiple trips to the loo and just generally feeling unwell.
All the cclassic symptoms of having diabetes. It wasn't until he finished a running session and ended up 50 yards behind his teammates
that the manager knew something had to be wrong, and sent him
to the doctor for tests.

One of his immediate thoughts was – will I be able to continue
with my soccer career and will I be able to play for England? As it
was all starting to sink in he made an offhand remark to his father
that he'd *'have to be the first diabetic to play for England'*.

He then asked the advice of three physicians, they all doubted it
was possible. Then he met a fourth physician, Dr Edwin Gale, who
believed he could. To this day, Gary still follows the advice of this
doctor.

He didn't give up, he learned how to cope, a lot of it through trial
and error and within three weeks of diagnosis he was donning his
soccer jersey. He has since gone on to become a full England International and lead a starring role, for 7 years as Captain of the First
Division Tottenham Hotspur Football team. One of the world's top
football clubs.

Gary realises that doctors can't predict what's going to happen to
us, that our bodies are going to be changing all of the time. Therefore we should take the necessary precautions and take heed of our
doctor's advice.

Bobby Robson, former England Football Manager, describes Gary
as 'the original Bionic Man'.

In 1994 Gary was awarded an MBE, Member of the British Em-
pire, by the Queen of England for services to football.

All of this has not come without hard work, dedication and above all commitment. He trains six days a week with Sundays off. During football season he plays up to three games per week.

Over the years he has amassed a strong following and reeives up to 50 fan letters per week. Hopefully this makes up for some of the abuse he receives on the pitch from the opposition fans. During one match in 1987, just as he was about to take a throw in, a fan from the opposing team threw a bag of sweets which hit him on the head. Some even go as far as yelling 'junkie' when he runs out onto the pitch. Football fans can be notoriously ruthless in their baiting of players. Gary shrugs it off by saying *'it's just part of the job'*.

After sixteen years of football and all of the daily rigours he puts his body through as a professional sportsman, Gary is a shining example that exercise and fitness are essential for people with diabetes.

Exercise, Endurance and the Person with Diabetes

Is success due to good physique, good psyche or good equipment?

Al Lewis, BSc, MSc, PhD
Professor, Oceanography & Zoology and Master Swimmer
University of British Columbia, Vancouver, BC, Canada

Exercise is considered to be activities beyond those required for daily routine responsibilities. For cardiovascular benefit, it should also be for an adequate length of time. Physique, of course, means physical or body structure and psyche is the spirit, soul and mind – or how a person mentally approaches exercise. The term equipment in the title is for the equipment that is used by the person who has diabetes whether it is for measuring blood glucose levels or exercising.

The benefits and values of an exercise programme for the person with diabetes can be improved by discussions with health care specialists – but only if the health care person appreciates the value of exercise. Unfortunately, one still finds health care specialists that do not believe exercise is valuable to the individual with diabetes. It is important for the health care person to realize that no matter the age of an individual, there is a need to find a proper exercise programme. This is to develop physiological as well as physical stature and, most importantly, the psyche that is needed to continue exercising.

Although there are many reasons why one might consider starting an exercise programme, enjoyment is essential for continuing to exercise. This enjoyment can include the pleasure of completing an exercise programme, the pleasure of improvement in the time to complete an event – or simply the joy of competing. Competition is really quite important to each of us, both over the short and long term. And the joy of competition can help push us a little harder, help us to improve both physically and mentally.

It is important to realize that competition need not be with others but only with ourselves, to improve our own ability and our confidence in our own abilities.

Success in exercising is often expressed by an improved outlook on the other things that we do – our work and our willingness to tackle the physical and mental problems that go with diabetes. Putting this into perspective with the title – the psyche of a person who has a suitable exercise programme is an indicator of the nature of an individual who is sincerely interested in properly maintaining his or her diabetic condition.

There are numerous problems for the person with diabetes who exercises. Unfortunately, these are often used as excuses rather than hurdles which must be overcome. The problems that must be addressed are problems from medication or the short – and long-term detrimental effects of the disease. They include both low and high blood glucose levels and the impact that they have during and after exercise programmes. It is important to realize that there are answers for most, if not all, problems. And these are answers that will allow each of us not only to exercise but to better participate in our day-to-day activities.

The equipment that we now have allows us to monitor blood glucose levels before and after exercise programmes. We can also do this during an exercise or event. Equipment will improve, not only in accuracy and reliability but also in ease of use. It is important to remember that although there may be good equipment, it is up to each of us to use it frequently enough and wisely enough to tell us what is happening to our blood glucose levels when the occasion requires. And to do this we must have a good deal of knowledge about our own diabetic profile.

Each of us needs to develop a fitness capable for what we want. We must have the proper mental attitude and the confidence. And we must be satisfied with what we are doing. These things can be obtained with today's equipment and a desire by each of us to improve our own physical and mental outlook on life. It is most important to recognize that diabetes must remain – simply – one additional hurdle in the path that each of us has chosen for our life.

Strength Training Basics

W. Guyton Hornsby, Jr, PhD, CDE, CSCS
Exercise Physiology, Division of Health Promotion
School of Physical Education, West Virginia University

Athletes know that strength is an essential quality for top performance in competitive sports. Unfortunately, athletes with diabetes may not be receiving the latest information on training for muscular strength and endurance. This presentation should provide you with a brief overview of how strength training programmes can be designed to help you achieve your individual fitness goals.

Training is able to increase strength in two fundamental ways: 1) by Muscle Recruitment – The nervous system can be trained to improve the way it calls on or recruits muscle fibers to contract and, 2) by Hypertrophy – Muscles can be trained to increase in size. Specific changes in the way the body functions are determined by the following variables of training: 1) Type, 2) Frequency, 3) Intensity, and 4) Duration of exercise.

To improve strength or muscular endurance, the type of exercise must involve working muscles against an appropriate resistive force. It makes little difference whether the resistance is provided by free weights using barbells or dumbbells, or by specialized machines such as those made by Nautilus or Universal. Regardless of the equipment chosen, it is important to learn proper lifting form.

Participants at the IDAA North American Conference were instructed in correct technique for the following basic free weight exercises: Squats, leg extensions, leg curls (for legs), bench press (chest), overhead press (shoulders), lat pulls (back), biceps curls and triceps extensions (arms), and curl-ups (abdominals). It may be helpful for you to work with a person certified as a strength and conditioning specialist (CSCS) by the National Strength and Conditioning Association. (For more information, contact NSCA at (402) 472–3000, U.S.A.)

Frequency of training should be two to three days per week for each muscle group. There should be at least 48 hours between workout sessions to allow for adequate recovery. You may simply choose to exercise all major muscle groups on a Monday, Wednesday, Friday schedule, or you may use a very advanced training schedule such as working your legs and chest on Monday and Thursday, shoulders and arms on Tuesday and Friday, and back and abdominals on Wednesday and Saturday.

The intensity of resistance exercise refers to how heavy you lift. This can be expressed in one of two ways: 1) In *absolute* terms as the actual load or amount of weight lifted, or 2) In *relative* terms as a percentage of your one repetition maximum (IRM). An IRM is the heaviest weight you can handle for one complete lift. For a strength training programme to be individualized, it is far better to think of the resistance as a *relative* intensity.

The duration of resistance exercise is best described in terms of volume or number of times you perform a particular lifting movement. Strength training is typically performed in three-six sets or groups of lifting movements repeated for a certain number of times. If you were to perform three sets of fifteen repetitions with 45 pounds in the bench press you would record this as $3 \times 15 \times 45$ lbs. The volume and the amount of rest you need between sets are very dependent on the intensity you select.

Intensity depends on the goals you are trying to achieve.

Local muscular endurance is developed by working with light loads (–40–70% IRM) for many repetitions (15–40 reps.) There will be little improvement in muscle recruitment with low intensity and muscle size is not increased until loads reach close to 60% IRM or greater. Using very light loads (50% IRM) produces limited gains in strength, but may be the best choice for people who have high blood pressure or other problems with their heart or blood vessels. These individuals may wish to use circuit weight training performing 8–10 different exercises for $3 \times 15 \times 40\%$ IRM with 30 seconds rest between sets.

Muscle recruitment is improved best by lifting very heavy weights (close to 90% IRM or greater). These heavy weights can obviously be lifted only a few times. A typical workout would include $3 \times 2 \times 95\%$ with three–five minutes rest between sets. Very intense lifting is associated with large increases in blood pressure. This type of lifting has been proven to be very effective for many athletes, and may be helpful for you, but you must be sure that you are free of complications of diabetes affecting the eyes or blood vessels.

Muscle hypertrophy is best developed by lifting moderately heavy weights (approximately 60–80% IRM) many times (5×10–15 with one–two minutes rest). These lighter weights allow for very high volume workouts and are popular with competitors in the sport of body building. While it is not uncommon to see a massive body builder pump out five or more sets in the bench press doing as many as 12–15 repetitions with 300 or more pounds, it is important to realize that this weight must be only moderately heavy for this individual athlete, otherwise they could not perform such a high number of repetitions.

A traditional way to train is by using resistances that are in between those used for recruitment and those used for hypertrophy. A typical example would be to perform three sets of five repetitions using a weight that is 85% of the IRM. It is often said that if a person selects only one intensity and duration of training, this would be the single best way to improve basic strength. The physiological effects are a moderate increase in muscle size with some improvement in neural recruitment.

Research has clearly shown however, that it is not best to always use only one intensity and duration for strength training. An athlete can maximize gains in hypertrophy and muscle recruitment only by varying the amount of weight used and number of sets and repetitions that are performed during different periods of training. This is commonly referred to as periodication.

Periodization training programmes are often used by athletes because they have found that variation is needed to make optimal gains in strength. Variation may also be important for people interested only in general fitness because it helps prevent boredom. The classic periodication programme contains four distinct training periods: 1) Hypertrophy, 2) Basic Strength, 3) Peaking, and 4) Active Rest. Each training period is approximately four weeks in length.

An athlete following the classic periodication model would begin by testing themselves for their IRM. If a person is new to weight training or if it is inadvisable to perform maximum lifts, a simple alternative is to select weights based on the Repetitions per Set model. For example, in the Hypertrophy period you would perform five sets of 10–15 reps with a weight that is 70% IRM, or a weight that allows you to do a maximum of 15 repetitions. This would be called your 15RM. From the diagram, you should be able to see that 70% IRM should provide a 15RM. You would perform 5 × 10–15 × 70% IRM, (or 15RM), with one–two minutes rest.

You would then start your Basic Strength period. This would be 3 × 5 × 85% IRM, or your 8RM. Rest during this period would be two–three minutes. If you are a competitive athlete and free of complications, you would then move to the Peaking period which uses very high intensity and low volume. Here you would do 3 × 2 × 95% IRM, or simply use your 3RM. Rest would be four–five minutes.

After you have completed 10–12 weeks of training, you would then enter the Active Rest period, where no weight training is performed. During this period you would do other activities such as jogging, basketball, or tennis. This Active Rest period is typically two–four weeks long and appears to be extremely effective in helping both the mind and body recover from intense training.

To be effective, a training programme must also be safe. People with diabetes should always check with their physician and work closely with their health care team to avoid any problems with exercise. For some people, strength training can be associated with potentially dangerous elevations in blood pressure. If you have complications of diabetes, you will need to find out what exercise intensities are appropriate for you.

Blood glucose responses to resistance exercise are also extremely important. The typical response to an intense weight training workout is a short-term rise in glucose, followed by a period which may last for many hours, where additional carbohydrate may be needed to prevent hypoglycemia. As with any exercise programme, glucose monitoring is the only way to know how your body responds.

There are other safety issues which apply to anyone lifting weights. Always warm-up and cool-down with exercise. The warm-up for lifting should be done in two stages. First, a 5–10 minute general warm-up period of aerobic exercise and stretching, followed by a specific warm-up in which you perform your lift with a very light weight to get the feel of the exercise.

Always use proper protective equipment including a lifting belt. Never hold your breath. Always continue to breathe, attempting to exhale while raising the weight and inhale while lowering the weight. You should always workout with a partner who knows how to spot you during your lifts.

There are many unanswered safety questions for people with diabetes who lift weights. Fortunately, the blanket statement that 'people with diabetes should never train with weights' is seldom heard any more. But we still do not know what intensities may be inappropriate for people with different complications, or if there are certain people who should not lift at all. At West Virginia University, we are currently conducting research studies to see how weight training affects blood flow and pressure in the eyes. Hopefully, with more scientific information we can safely design strength training programs that allow athletes with diabetes to maximize their potential.

How to Begin a Training Programme in Swimming

Al Lewis, PhD
Master Swimmer
Diabetes – 54 years

First answer these questions:

1   How much time will I devote to working out?
    20 minutes a day?
    60 minutes?
    More than 60 minutes per day?
    1 time a week?
    3 times a week?
    More than 3 times per week?
2   Is my schedule flexible or rigid?
    Am I a morning or evening person?
    What time of day fits me and my schedule?
3   How long has it been since I've had a physical?
    What is my doctor's recommendation on exercise for me at this time?
4   What are my goals or reasons for starting this programme?
    Fitness?
    Weight loss?
    State or national record times?
    Open water swims?
    Any combination of the above?
5   What is my level of fitness before starting the swimming programme?

After answering these questions, make up a schedule that is reasonable for your age, time commitments, goals and personality.

Next make up a diary or chart so that you can keep track of the time spent training, type and duration of exercise and finally progress toward your goals.

The following paragraphs will give you examples of both the diary/chart concept and planned workouts to get you started on your way to fitness, fun and friendship.

These progressions are suggestions, not rigid guidelines. Adjust them, change them or just use them to help you set up your own programme.

People will progress at different rates, depending on the starting point. One caution; many folks start out with great enthusiasm and purpose, blow your energy, become discouraged and drop out of the programme after just a short time. Keep your competitive drive in check, start slowly, increase the work load gradually and enjoy your programme and efforts year in and year out.

Most programmes recommend workouts lasting 45 minutes to 1½ hours, 3 to 5 times a week.

A beginning programme as suggested by the National Masters Swim Committee is:

First 2 weeks:	100 yards each day in four swims of 25 yards (mts)
2nd–6th week:	200 yards each day in two swims of 100 yards (mts)
6th–16th week:	400 yards each day in four swims of 100 yards (mts)
16th–24th week:	600 yards each day in three swims of 200 yards (mts)
24th–32nd week:	800 yards each day in either four swims of 200 yards (mts) or two swims of 400 yards each
At 32 weeks:	At least 800 yards a day either as eight 100 yards, four 200 yards, two 400 yards or one 800 yard swims
Thereafter:	Any type of workout you are physically able to perform.

The method of identifying the distance of the workout can be expressed in a number of ways as shown in the examples below.

SAMPLE WORKOUT

1 16 lengths – P crawl (P – using arms only)
   4 lengths – IM (one length each fly, back, breast, crawl)
  16 lengths – 2 back, 2 breast, 2 free, 2 fly, repeat
   4 lengths – IM
   4 lengths – easy (cool down)
  44 lengths total

2 24 lengths – warm up 12 crawl, 3 fly, 3 back, 3 breast, 3 choice
  16 lengths – 2 P each back & breast, 4 P crawl
   8 lengths – fin K: 2 fly, 2 back, 2 crawl, 2 fly
   4 lengths – IM
   8 lengths – easy
  60 lengths total

3   2 minutes easy swim
     15 min. S weakest stroke, not crawl
     10 min. K choice
     15 min. S favourite stroke
     <u>2 min. cool down</u>
     44 min. total

4   1 × 400 warm up
     3 × 400 descending rest 30 seconds between 400's
     8 × 25 at 75% working heart rate
     8 × 100 – alternating 100 IM and 100 P choice
     8 × 25 on 30 seconds
     8 × Dive and 5 strokes at race pace
     <u>200 easy</u>
3000 mts +

WARMUPS AND SWIM-DOWNS
Why they are important

The warmup is a time to work the cardiovascular system, muscles, joints and mind progressively from a slow to medium pace without traumatizing any or all of the parts.

Seven good reasons to warm up for a sports competition or workout:

1 Heart and lung function is gradually accelerated thus reducing the risk of electrical or chemical dysfunction in the heart. The dysfunction can be caused by a sudden change, from rest to high demand, that will occur without a warmup.

2 The rate of oxygen transfer from blood to tissues and carbon dioxide from tissues to blood is increased, thus increasing the work capacity of muscles.

3 With each 1 degree increase in muscle temperature there is a 13% increase in metabolic rate. Among other things, this helps the nervous system to become sensitized to hard physical work. This improves reflex action and coordination. Working muscles will contract and relax at a faster rate and antagonistic muscles will relax more.

4 Body temperatures rise and warmup exercises also cause fatty material in tendons to become 'oily', thus improving the muscle's mechanical efficiency and performance through decreased tendon-muscle friction.

5. The higher body temperatures and increased efficiency and elas-

ticity of muscles (from static stretching exercise) increases the range of motion and reduces the risk of muscle soreness and injury, particularly around the joints.

6   The body and mind are given a low intensity rehearsal of the motions to be performed in full later.

7   Warmups work out physical bugs and tensions – sort of clearing the physiological and psychological deck – to get ready to perform with a clear mind.*

The warmup also helps answer 'How am I feeling today, what is my body telling me?', 'What kind of feedback am I getting?', 'Am I really doing this because I'd rather be on the golf course?', 'Do I want to work out, am I ready for 3000 meters?'. Your heart rate will be the key to many of these enquiries.

Many warmups are made up of:

1   Stretching exercises on land.
2   Slow swimming at 50 to 60 percent of the 'Working Heart Rate' (WHR) for 200–400 meters (yards) using long, stretching strokes.
3   Kicking and pulling up to 200 meters.
4   If at a meet – two or three 25's at 85% of race pace and some starts from the blocks. Remember to check out the turn flags if you are a backstroker.
    Total warmup distance = 200–800 meters (yards).

SWIMDOWN – COOLDOWN
The reverse of the warmup

The cooldown helps the body systems slow down gradually. This will help to minimize the sore and aching muscles by eliminating lactic acid build-up resulting from extensive exercising.

This part of the workout includes:

1   A 3 to 10 minute swim at 50% speed, thus allowing the heart rate to slow to near its resting rate.
2   Reviewing drills at a slow pace.
3   Stretching exercises on land, much the same as in the warmup.

* Modified from the *Sungod Aquatic Centre Fitness 1111 Brochure* (Delta, British Columbia, February 1987)

Ski Instruction . . . The Real Story

Brian DuBoff*

It's funny the way some jobs have reputations associated with them that usually have nothing at all to do with reality. Case in point: the Ski Instructor. Sure, the job has its memorable moments, but Hollywood has not told the whole truth (amazing, huh!). A full winter day on the side of a Vermont mountain teaching, inspiring and entertaining groups of 6–16 people, under the best of circumstances, is a constant mental and physical challenge. The circumstances are rarely ideal with temperatures dropping down into the single digits, adults with absolutely no athletic ability who become either stiff as boards or limp as rag dolls, and teens who only want to race down the expert terrain. As instructor, my three goals for any class are safety, fun, and learning for each and every student regardless of the intra-group diversity. If the first two goals are achieved, the third usually 'just happens.' Control and trust are major issues when guiding a group of strangers into a potentially dangerous situation. Control and trust are the same issues I face when considering my own Type I diabetes in light of this leadership role.

I've had diabetes for 16 years and for the last 5–6 years now I've been on an intensive insulin plan that has worked out really well for me. Sometimes referred to as the 'poor man's pump,' I take a human Regular (Actrapid) insulin before each meal, and a beef/pork Ultralente insulin at bedtime. If necessary, I supplement extra Regular insulin as needed using a sliding scale. Frequent glucose monitoring is the key to success with this intensive routine, ranging from three to ten times a day. Because the beef/pork Ultralente is the longest lasting and least 'peaky' available, I can take it once a day. I choose before bedtime (11.30 pm) in order to ensure even absorption and because this gives me one last chance to supplement with Regular if needed, and to get things under control. In addition, this allows me to carry only Regular insulin and my meter with me all day in my ski suit. Using the Novo/Nordisk Regular pen cartridges as 'mini bottles' with an insulin syringe is a real space

* Brian DuBoff has a MS degree in Scientific Administration. He lives in Burlington, VT and works as a ski instructor at Smugglers' Notch Ski Resort in Jeffersonville, VT. Each summer he teaches in-line skating and is a founding member of RollVermont, an in-line skating event raising money for diabetes research through the ADA Vermont Affiliate.

saver. Both fit into my Exactech meter case nicely, providing a complete day kit in the size of an eye glass case.

Each day begins at 6.45 am with a finger-stick, a shot of Regular (Actrapid), breakfast, and an hour drive to the mountain. Arriving at 8.30 am I would test again, supplement (food or insulin) if necessary, dress appropriately (including extra batteries for my boot heaters-equipment as important for me as skis and gloves), check my carbohydrate supply (fast acting glucose and a mix of granola, string cheese and fig newtons), and race out to the first of five ski school line-ups. We hold one hour private lessons at 9 am, 12 noon and 3 pm, and 1 3/4 hour group lessons at 1.15 am and 1.30 pm. Two group lessons were guaranteed Monday through Friday, but private lessons were not assured. Usually people sign up for private lessons in the middle and at the end of the week. What this means to me is that some days are significantly more active than others. Most Mondays and Tuesdays are just group lessons with free time or skiing in between, while the second half of the week could include between two and five lessons a day with very little time for testing and eating.

Because the instructors' room is a major hike from the line-up area, I stash lunch in the lift hut and insulin (with a syringe) in a pocket. If I get a noon private lesson I typically dose and gobble before the 1.30 pm group. Testing is not usually necessary by 1 pm since telltale signs of hypoglycemia begin to surface. Alternatively, if there is no 12 noon private lesson I opt for a more leisurely test/dose/munch back in the instructors' room and take a few runs before the second group line-up. At the end of the day I test one more time before driving home. At the beginning of the season this final blood check was not a hard and fast rule, but too many times my blood sugar level was way too high by dinner time. It seemed like a good idea.

I never hid my diabetes while teaching and would usually explain why I was eating strange looking candy and not offering some to the whole class. Whenever a physician sat next to me on the lift I would go into my public-service mode and make sure she/he was current on their diabetes treatment skills. One day my supervisor introduced me to a family whose 11 year old son had diabetes and was in the children's programme. The father introduced himself as a physician and explained to me that Jonathon had actually been diagnosed *three weeks earlier!* I was very impressed with how these people were committed to living their lives, even if it meant sharing it with diabetes. My girlfriend, Erin, who also has Type I diabetes, happened to be skiing that day and we all sat down for a couple of hours at the end of the day and talked shop. Questions were asked and opinions offered. Jonathon patiently listened as the expert diabetic skiers carried on and on about their own successes and failures. As the conversation ended it was clear to me that the issues of control and trust also existed between the parents and son. How they chose to deal with diabetes-related issues will most certainly have long-lasting advantageous effects.

In terms of my ski instructing and my diabetes control, they are either completely related or unrelated. What I mean is that if I take good care of my diabetes, I can take good care of my class. In a sense, my diabetes does not impact upon my ability to instruct – they are unrelated. If, however, my diabetes gets out of control (a severe hypoglycemic reaction for example), class is interrupted and my trustworthiness to lead the group through a difficult situation comes under question. They are definitely related. How these issues are dealt with determine their impact.

Skiing is like life. You start out on the baby slope falling down a lot. You get better and go faster and fall down less often. Soon you try skiing the expert slopes and you're falling down constantly. You get better and go faster and fall down less often. Life is full of moguls and patches of ice constantly challenging our trust and control. How these issues are dealt with determine their impact.

A Unique Study Takes People with Diabetes to New Depths

Gary Scheiner
Countdown Magazine
Juvenile Diabetes Foundation

Twenty years ago, an active person diagnosed with diabetes was likely to hear the same words over and over again: *'I'm sorry, but you can't do that.'* Much has changed in the last two decades. With advances in applied research, bio-engineering, and self-care practices (such as blood glucose monitoring), people with diabetes can achieve just about anything. From the highest ranks of professional sports to 'adventure' activities, people with diabetes everywhere are doing things no one would have expected.

DEEP-SIXED?

Historically, people with diabetes have had problems obtaining certification for scuba diving due to the risks associated with underwater insulin reactions. Some organizations, including the YMCA and the National Association of Underwater Instructors (NAUI), simply will not certify anyone with insulin-dependent diabetes due to associated risks. Others, including the Professional Association of Diving Instructors (PADI) and Handicap Scuba Association, require a minimum of written medical consent and instructor approval before training can begin.

Technically, no organization can prohibit a person from scuba diving, but essential training can and has been withheld based on a person's status as an insulin-dependent diabetic patient.

According to experts, the skepticism is not unfounded. With most dives lasting an average of 30 to 40 minutes, the possibility of developing hypoglycemia while under water is significant – especially for novice divers who may be nervous and expend a great deal more energy than is necessary. Even experienced divers run a risk if they're not careful. It takes a minute or two of steady, coordinated action in order to resurface, so a person with typical symptoms of hypoglycemia (shakiness, confusion) may have a very hard time getting out of the water. The results, obviously, could be disastrous.

More than 100 diving-related deaths are reported each year, at least some of which are suspected to be related to diabetes, according to the Divers Alert Network.

DETERMINED TO DIVE

Steve Prosterman, IDAA member, diving and field supervisor at the University of the Virgin Islands Marine Science Center in St Thomas, V.I., has had insulin-dependent diabetes since childhood. Determined not to let his disease stand in the way of his love for the ocean, he has been scuba diving for almost 20 years.

Prosterman recognized that one of the reasons for all the skepticism was the fact that no quantifiable research or established protocols existed for making diving safe for people with diabetes. With this in mind, and with support from the University of the Virgin Islands Marine Science Center, he set out to develop a series of guidelines that would minimize many of the hazards associated with scuba diving. Those guidelines were later presented at the National Underwater Conference, sponsored by NAUI in October 1992.

Some of the recommendations are listed below. According to Prosterman, many of them can be applied to a number of activities in which a person with insulin-dependent diabetes may find himself or herself isolated for any significant length of time.

- Do not dive when glycemic control is generally poor. Hyperglycemia, as well as hypoglycemia, can impair one's ability to perform safely in the water.

- Monitor blood sugar levels four times (one hour before the dive, half an hour before, immediately prior and immediately after) in order to determine:
1 the blood sugar level prior to the dive;
2 the direction and stability of the glucose level (is it going up, down, or not changing?);
3 how the dive affected blood sugar levels (for future adjustments).

Blood sugar should be slightly above normal prior to diving –8.3 mmol/l+ if rising and 10 mmol/l– if stable (but without ketones). If the blood sugar level is falling or is below these levels, the person should not dive without eating some extra carbohydrate and rechecking to see that the level has been stabilized.

- The depth of dives should be limited to no more than 60 feet in order to avoid 'nitrogen narcosis' – a deep water condition that often masks or mimics symptoms of hypoglycemia.

- Develop an underwater communication system (via hand signals) to let a partner know if low blood sugar is developing. It will be essential to know the signs/symptoms of hypoglycemia as well as how to treat it.

In Prosterman's study, the dive was terminated immediately upon signs of hypoglycemia. The whole group surfaced, and sugar was administered in the form of 'InstaGlucose' tubes.

'It doesn't work to just go out and scuba dive', explained George Burghen, MD, chief of Endocrinology and Metabolism at the University of Tennessee, and a colleague in Prosterman's research efforts. 'You really have to understand your body before trying something like this. Monitoring blood sugar helps build in a "safety factor" and is the best way to learn how your body responds to different types of activities.'

Prosterman agreed, 'Monitoring is definitely the key. By keeping a close watch on blood sugar levels and the direction they are headed, people with diabetes can do just about anything.'

THINK BEFORE YOU SINK

The scuba diving study demonstrates an important point – it is OK for people with diabetes to push themselves and strive for new heights (or depths) as long as they are responsible about it. Common sense dictates that any activity that isolates a diabetic individual for an extended period of time – whether it be sailing on a lake, climbing the side of a mountain or pedalling down a country road – requires some extra planning and precautions. That means blood sugar monitoring at regular intervals, carrying extra food, wearing medical identification and bringing along change for a phone or vending machine.

hiness to lead the group through a difficult situation
question. They are definitely related. How these is-
with determine their impact.

e life. You start out on the baby slope falling down a
etter and go faster and fall down less often. Soon you

BDA Holidays

The British Diabetic Association offer numerous events, forums and courses for individuals with diabetes and their families. These events provide an excellent backdrop for learning and socialising. They all involve a dedicated team of volunteers and medical staff to put everyone's mind at ease.

In 1990 I was involved with the annual Youth Diabetes (YD) Project held in Firbush, Scotland, organized by Dr Ray Newton. The YD Project was founded by Professor Jim Farquhar in hopes of uniting people with diabetes in a fun, relaxed atmosphere and to help them learn and share their experiences of living with diabetes. All I can say is that I wish I'd been introduced to this type of holiday years ago. I made some great new friends, learnt more about my diabetes and about myself and tried my hand at a lot of new sports. What you can learn from a week on this holiday is more valuable than reading any textbook on diabetes.

Some other events brought to you by the British Diabetic Association are: Family Weekends; Parent Network Events; Parent Link Course; BDA Teen Weekends; the infamous YD Conference (an annual weekend event held at Birmingham University); and Teenage Holidays including skiing in the Northern French Alps; Outward Bound in Wales; activities in Loch Lomond, Scotland where you can play volley ball, archery, windsurfing, canoeing and try some gorge walking.

Glossary

Abbreviations:

BG:	also known as blood sugar or blood glucose
CARBOS:	carbohydrates
HYPERS:	hyperglycaemia
HYPOS:	hypoglycaemia

Autonomic Neuropathy: damage to the system of nerves which regulate many autonomic functions of the body such as stomach emptying, sexual function (potency) and blood pressure control.

Carbohydrates: a class of food which comprises starches and sugars and is most readily available in the body for energy. Found mainly in plant foods. Examples are rice, bread, potatoes, pasta, dried beans.

Control: usually refers to blood glucose control. The aim of good control is to achieve normal blood glucose levels, 4–7 mmol/l.

Glucose: form of sugar made by the digestion of carbohydrates. Absorbed into the bloodstream where it circulates and is used for energy.

Glycogen: the form in which carbohydrate is stored in the liver. It is often known as animal starch.

Hormone: substance generated in one gland or organ which is carried by the blood to another part of the body to stimulate another organ into activity.

Hyperglycaemia: high blood glucose or blood sugar, above 10 mmol/l.

Hypoglycaemia: low blood glucose or blood sugar, below 3 mmol/l.

Insulin: a hormone produced by the beta cells of the pancreas and responsible for the control of blood glucose. Insulin can only be given by injection because the digestive juices destroy its action if taken by mouth.

Insulin Reaction: another name for hypoglycaemia or a hypo. In America it is called an insulin shock or shock.

Intramuscular: a deep injection into the muscle.

Ketoacidosis: a serious condition due to lack of insulin which results in body fat being used up to form ketones and acids. Characterised by high blood glucose levels, ketones in the urine, vomiting, drowsiness, heavy laboured breathing and a smell of acetone on the breath.

Ketones: acid substances formed when body fat is used up to provide energy.

Nephropathy: kidney damage. In the first instance this makes the kidney more leaky so that albumin appears in the urine. At a later stage it may affect the function of the kidney and in severe cases lead to kidney failure.

Neuropathy: damage to the nerves. This may be peripheral or autonomic (see peripheral neuropathy and autonomic neuropathy). It can occur with diabetes especially when poorly controlled, but also has other causes.

Peripheral Neuropathy: damage to the nerves supplying the muscles and skin. This can result in diminished sensation, particularly in the feet and legs, and in muscle weakness.

Retina: light sensitive coat at the back of the eye.

Retinopathy: damage to the retina.

Urinalysis: analysis of a sample of urine.

Copied by permission from Dr Charles Fox, co-author of the reference book *Diabetes At Your Fingertips*, Class Publishing. Incidentally, this is the best reference book on the market, one I refer to on numerous occasions.

Useful Addresses

Advanced Care Products
PO Box 106, Ipswich,
Suffolk IP6 9EF

Bayer Plc (Ames Division)
Evans House, Hamilton Close,
Houndmills, Basingstoke,
Hampshire RG21 2YE

Becton Dickinson UK Limited
Between Towns Road,
Cowley, Oxford OX4 3LY

British Association of
Counselling
37a Sheep Street, Rugby,
Warwickshire CV21 3BX

British Diabetic Association
10 Queen Anne Street,
London W1M 0BD

Boehringer Mannheim UK
Bell Lane, Lewes,
East Sussex BN7 1LG

Bristol-Myers Squibb
Pharmaceuticals Limited
141–149 Staines Road,
Hounslow, Middlesex TW3 3JA

Eating Disorders Association
Sackville Place,
44 Magdalen Street,
Norwich NR3 1JU

Eli Lilly and Company Limited
Dextra Court, Chapel Hill,
Basingstoke,
Hampshire RG21 2SY

International Diabetic Athletes
Association (Head Office)
6829 N. 12th Street,
Suite 205,
Phoenix, Arizona,
U.S.A. 85014

Kellogg's Company of Great
Britain Limited
The Kellogg Building,
Talbot Road,
Manchester M16 0PU

Lifescan – Division of Ortho
Diagnostic Systems Ltd.
Enterprise House,
Station Road, Loudwater,
High Wycombe,
Bucks HP10 9UF

MediSense Britain Limited
PO Box 2159, Coleshill,
Birmingham B46 1HZ

Novo Nordisk Pharmaceuticals
Limited
Novo Nordisk House,
Broadfields Park,
Brighton Road,
Pease Pottage, Crawley,
West Sussex RH11 9RT

P.R. (Cooper) Footline Ltd
Sycamore Works,
Tilton on the Hill,
Leicestershire LE7 9LG

Ulverscroft Large Print Books
The Green, Bradgate Road,
Anstey, Leicester LE7 7FU

Acknowledgements

The author wishes to acknowledge the following companies
for their encouragement and support:
Andy Ripley & Espree – The Club, Fitness Management
Abbott Laboratories Ltd
Advanced Care Products Ltd
Bayer (Ames Division) plc
Baxter Health Care
Becton Dickinson UK Limited
Bio-Rad Laboratories Ltd
Boehringer Mannheim UK
Braun Medical Ltd
Bristol-Myers Squibb Pharmaceuticals Limited
British Diabetic Association
CAMP Limited
Capel-Cure Myers Capital Management Limited
Cereal Partners U.K.
CliniMed Ltd
ConvaTec Limited
CPC (United Kingdom) Limited (Dextro Energy Tablets)
Crookes Healthcare Ltd (Sweetex)
Eli Lilly and Company Limited
Esso Research Centre and Mr Roger Park
Gainor Medical Europe Limited
HNE Healthcare
Hermes Sweeteners (UK) Limited
Hoechst UK Limited
Huntleigh Technology plc
Hypoguard (UK) Ltd
Invicta Pharmaceuticals
Janssen Research Foundation
Kellogg's Company of Great Britain Limited
Knoll Limited
Lifescan – Division of Ortho Diagnostics Systems Ltd
Lloyds Chemist plc
MediSense Britain Limited

Mentor Medical Systems Ltd
Morning Foods Ltd (Mornflake)
Novo Nordisk Pharmaceuticals Limited
P.R. Cooper (Footline) Ltd
Pharma-Plast Ltd
Roussel Laboratories Limited
Sandoz Pharmaceuticals (UK) Limited
Scientific Hospital Supplies (Juvela) UK Limited
Scientific Laboratory Supplies Ltd
Scotia Pharmaceuticals Ltd
Servier Laboratories Ltd
Seven Seas Health Care Limited
Shalcombe Manor & Colonel Ken McKenzie Walker
Sherwood Medical Industries Ltd
Specialist Services (Scotland) Ltd
St Ivel Ltd
Sterling Health Limited
Streamline Foods
Thorntons plc
Thursday Cottage Ltd
Ulverscroft Large Print Books Limited
Upjohn Limited
YSI Limited
and to thank the following individuals for their time and expertise in reviewing the manuscript and offering constructive criticism and advice:
Dr Charles Fox, Sister Joan Allwinkle, Dr Jill Challener, Dr Chris Gillespie, Dr David Leslie, Alison McKay, Joy McLeod, Sister Diane Slater, Alison Strawford, Kate Thomas, Rosamund Snow (and her mom!), Deborah Tully, Thomas Mulholland and all the authors of contributing articles and a special thank you to Tina Ryan.

Index

CONTENTS